My Interesting Life

The Adventures of an Itinerant Corn Cutter

by

Evan F. Meltzer, DPM (retired)

My Interesting Life The Adventures of an Itinerant Corn Cutter
©2024 Evan F. Meltzer

All rights reserved.

ISBN: 9798795302416

Dedication

I dedicate this memoir to my wife and partner throughout this journey, Linda Blazek Meltzer. Without her support, encouragement, sense of adventure, creative thinking and love, we might still be living in Ithaca (or somewhere in the Caribbean) and would have missed out on this interesting life.

The 1970s song by Gerry Rafferty, "Right Down the Line," describes better than I could what Linda's support meant to me for all these years.

Table of Contents

Dedication
Author's Note 1
Preface 3
Introduction 5
Chapter One New York, The Land of Taxes 11
Chapter Two New Mexico, Land of Enchantment 49
Chapter Three Fort Hood, America's Hammer 87
Chapter Four Montana, The Last Best Place 109
Chapter Five Is it Hampton, Jackson, or San Diego? 191
Chapter Six Mississippi, The Magnolia State 205
Chapter Seven Return to Texas, The Alamo City 221
Chapter Eight Final Thoughts 229
About the Author 233
Acknowledgments 235

Author's Note

The title of this memoir comes from the early history of podiatry as we know it today.

In Europe in the Middle Ages, there were vendors who traveled between villages carrying wooden tool boxes that contained crude cutting instruments. Something like shoeshine vendors of today, these early traveling "corn cutters" would set up their tool box and holler, "Corns to pick, corns to pick." Folks needing their services would place their foot on top of the tool box or the knee, and the chiropodist (precursor name for podiatrist) would then proceed to take care of the presented calloused tissue. It was strictly a cash business. Fortunately for them, health insurance companies and the Occupational Safety and Health Administration (OSHA) had not yet been established.

The surnames mentioned in the introduction are real names. With a few exceptions, the names in the text of this memoir have been changed to protect the innocent- and the guilty!

Preface

Anyone who writes a memoir must have a reason to write their story. I believe my life has taken a different course from many of my Baby Boomer contemporaries. I have mostly taken the high road in life. I attribute most of my life choices to the constant exposure at an impressionable age to the principles promoted by the Boy Scouts of America. I was brainwashed in a good way after attending scout meetings every Monday night during the school year for seven years. I learned much later in my life that the Mormon Church was one of the biggest supporters of this organization. I believe that I may have taken these principles to heart to a greater degree than many of my generation, although I am not a Mormon. I guess I matured from a Boy Scout into a "Man Scout." Exactly how does a kid growing up in Rochester, New York live in Mississippi after moving from Michigan, Colorado, Pennsylvania, Maryland, New Mexico, Texas, and Montana?

I remain physically distant but emotionally close with my son, Peter. I asked my estranged daughter once, "Wendy, why do you hate me so much?" She told me to my face, "I don't hate you Dad, you are just not a part of my life." This is her choice, although she is no doubt the remaining casualty of a divisive divorce from her mother. You will see glimpses of my "Not being a part of her life" in the following pages. Perhaps another reason to document my story is to share it with them some day if they are interested. Mainly

I believe this is an exercise in self-discovery. I also enjoy writing and editing, and had been a reviewer for a professional peer reviewed journal in foot and ankle surgery.

Early in my life I became fascinated by the scientific world; specifically in rocks and minerals. This interest naturally led to the study of the makeup of these specimens, hence the early pursuit of chemistry and physics. Learning about the localities of these specimens spurned my interest in travel from watching the seductive slide shows of Western locales shown by the late Bill Pinch (williampinch.com); to making field trips with my family and others, including several trips with Bill, to collect them for myself. I did not pursue the study of the biological and medical sciences until much later.

There are sentinel moments in everyone's life where choices are made that profoundly affect the direction of one's life. I hope to revisit these moments in my life in the pages that follow and examine why I made the choices I did. Through a self-discovery course I took in the late 1990's, I learned that my true calling in life was to be a healer and educator.

When I shared this epiphany with my late lifelong friend, Dr. Richard Erenstone of Lake Placid, New York while riding a chair lift together at Whiteface Mountain, I thought he would fall off the lift from laughter. "You spent how much on that course to find that out? I could have told you that for free". Dick, who was a well-respected optometrist, had always been a very goal-oriented individual who had the same intensity of scouting exposure as I had. We both became Eagle Scouts from the same troop. It seems there was little in his life that ever mystified him. How the lives of Bill, Dick and others affected my life will be explored in the pages that follow.

INTRODUCTION

I was born in the fifth month of the first year of the Baby Boom era.

The day of my birth, also happened to be Mother's Day. Every seven years while my mother was alive, I celebrated the dual events of my birthday and Mother's Day with my parents.

My mother's obstetrician called me the eight pound ten ounce "blond bomber" due to my size and the shock of blond hair I had at birth. I was delivered at the University of Rochester's renowned Strong Memorial Hospital. I am a proud member of the vanguard class of baby boomers that also include the former presidents George W. Bush, July 6th and Bill Clinton, August 19th.

My mother, Shirley Gold Meltzer was born on February 14, 1923, the younger daughter of Ethel Finer Gold and Louis Jacob Gold (a World War I veteran). My father Harold Meltzer (a World War II veteran) was born on September 29, 1921, one of five children of Rebecca Feinberg Meltzer and Leonard Meltzer. My sister, Sherry Jean Meltzer Gold (wife of Morrie Gold, MD, also from Rochester) was born on October 22, 1948.

My grandfather Leonard Meltzer was born in Radescevicz, Belarus in 1892. That village no longer exists, but its name is proudly etched into the glass windows along with the names of other extinct Eastern European communities that line the skybridge at the United States Memorial Holocaust Museum in Washington, D.C.

At the time of my birth, my parents were living in an apartment on Hollenbeck Street in Rochester, above a dairy, and within sight of a small manufacturing business named the Haloid Company. That business would eventually become known as the Xerox Corporation.

I attended the Rochester public schools, graduating twenty-fifth out of five hundred fellow seniors from East High School in 1964. I then attended Michigan State University where I graduated with my bachelor's degree in Chemistry. I worked the summers of my college years in Rochester for "The Great Yellow Father", aka the Eastman Kodak Company. Working at Kodak was a learning experience in several ways.

I worked what was called "swing shift" in the Paper Service Division. One week I worked eight to four, followed the next week's shift from four to midnight, and the following week the "graveyard" shift was midnight to eight. "Lunch break" on that shift was usually at four a.m. I really couldn't eat much at that hour. One of my co-workers worked that shift exclusively for twenty years! I worked all shifts in a darkroom so that the photographic paper being manufactured was exposed to test colors in the darkroom, inserted into an automatic developing device by us and examined by supervisors in a lighted part of the test area for quality control.

This type of factory work really made me appreciate my college education that would give me the tools to get a white-collar job after graduation. My least favorite shift was four to midnight. I was working when all my friends were partying. In its heyday, Kodak employed one out of every four workers in the Rochester area. For many years, Kodak was the prime sponsor of the world-famous Albuquerque International Balloon Fiesta. More photographs were supposedly taken at this event than any other single event in the world. As digital photography became commonplace, other sponsors such as Canon became the main sponsors. In 2020 the Kodak workforce was forty-five hundred, about a ninety percent decrease from when I last worked there in 1967. The population of Rochester is now only about two-thirds of what it was when I lived there.

From East Lansing, Michigan, I traveled to Boulder, Colorado where I attended graduate school at the University of Colorado. I left Boulder in 1970 with my Master's degree in Biochemistry. I then moved to Canton, New York where I taught organic chemistry and physical science from 1970-1973 at the State University of New York's two-year college there.

I then moved to the Philadelphia, PA area in 1973 to begin my podiatry studies at Temple University. I was supported with an Army Health Professions Scholarship to fund my four-year education at Temple. I am again grateful to my friend, Dick Erenstone, who told me about the Army Scholarship program that changed the course of my life.

After graduating with my doctorate in podiatry in 1977, I entered Active Duty in the Army as a podiatrist at Fort Meade, Maryland. I was honorably discharged in 1982 and began private practice. I lived and practiced in Ithaca, New York until 2001, and this is where my life really gets interesting.

Chapter One includes vignettes of various events in New York leading up to the eventual move from that state. During this time, my wife Linda and I have moved from New York to New Mexico, followed by moves to Texas, Montana, Mississippi and back to Texas. We spent all but five months apart from October 2005-September 2007; Linda in Texas and me working in Montana.

The first three words in M. Scott Peck's landmark book, *The Road Less Traveled,* are: "Life is difficult."

Well, there is difficult and then there's ridiculous! For the tax year 2007, my CPA filed tax returns for three states in addition to the federal return. It would have been four states, but Texas has no state income tax. Even this experienced accountant was challenged by the complexities of our life.

This is a story of adventure, travel, unexpected professional disappointments, perseverance and determination. A doctor's life is often romanticized as a life of wealth and status, free from the ordinary politics of the workplace. My memoir of this time reveals the true underbelly of life as a government-employed doctor. You will also get an insider's view of what it was like to live through a medical malpractice trial and the subsequent effect on a doctor's professional life.

Throughout the trials and tribulations of this part of my life, I feel richer for the experience and value my journey. I've learned about the ways of conservative Southern Baptists in Mississippi and about the true meaning of what mañana really means in New Mexico.

I understand what a Montana wheat farmer means when he says, "I'm taking my rig on the High Line."

I definitely know where bread comes from.

I know that a Southern gal was talking to me alone when she says, "Ya'll have a nice day." The first time I heard that phrase, I turned around to see who else she was referring to.

I understand what a "Good ole Boy" was after meeting Billy Bob and Jimmy Ray. I've learned that chitlins, greens and mudbugs are edible. I've also learned to ask folks in Mississippi, "How's your mamma."

I've met James Smith and his brother Jimmy.

At the Jackson, Mississippi VA, a female veteran came to my clinic, and I asked her, "How can I help you today?"

She said, "I have Arthur."

I asked, "Is he with you now?"

"He's always with me, I have Arthur-itis."

A condition described in this state as a condition that affects the joints. And I thought that "Arthur" was the name of a childhood friend and also that of my father's younger brother!

I was also once asked a question in Browning, Montana that I doubt I will ever be asked again, "How were your Indian Days?"

I was invited to a sweat lodge.

I have always been fascinated by local surnames and regional accents. Growing up in New York State, my friends, relatives, co-workers and classmates had surnames like Kehrer, Woerner, Hudnut, Eberlein, Angelico, Caviccioli, Capaldo, Lukasiewicz, Lambiase, Glicken, Stoler, Dinaburg, Chernow, Ouderkirk and Uhorchak. These surnames reflect the great American melting pot of immigrants who passed through Ellis Island and settled in New York State. One name (Hudnut) was a direct descendant of the Mayflower Pilgrims.

The Land of Enchantment's license plate identifies itself as "New Mexico USA, lest it is ever confused with our Southern neighbor, Mexico. It's the land of Martinez, Chavez, Gallegos, Galindo, Gabaldon, Lujan, Begay, and Yazzie.

The Big Sky country of Montana on the Blackfeet Indian reservation is the home of Tail Feathers, Spotted Eagle, Rides at the Door, Young Running Crane, Arrow Top Knot, Heavyrunner, Bearmedicine, Bullcalf, Kickingwoman, Makes Cold Weather and my favorite, Prairie Chicken Shoe.

White bread and vanilla-flavored Central Texas was home to Smith, Jones, Johnson, Brown, Davis and Harris.

Mississippi was home to folks with surnames like McGehee, Moak, Herrin, Breeland, Foshee, Fortenberry and their Texas cousins Smith, Jones, Johnson, Brown, Davis and Harris.

Some names are even backwards. In New York, they would be Gary Wister, Stuart Sharkey and Virgil Torrance. In Mississippi they're really Wister Gary, Sharkey Stuart, and Torrance Virgil.

I know that others move around and have many jobs, but I feel mine is a unique adventure and I hope you ("Ya'll") enjoy sharing it with me through the pages that follow.

Chapter One

New York, The Land of Taxes

(Also known as The Empire State)
1982-2001

I was born in the first year of the baby boom era and lived in Rochester, New York until 1964. I enjoyed my extended family including both grandparents and all my aunts, uncles and cousins on both sides of the family. The Meltzer side gradually moved away as their vocations took them to other locations.

As already mentioned in my introduction, after graduating from East High School, I attended Michigan State University from 1964-1968 and graduated in 1968 with a degree in chemistry. I continued my graduate studies at the University of Colorado-Boulder from 1968-1970 where I received a master's degree in Biochemistry. From 1970-1973, I lived in frigid Canton, New York where I taught organic chemistry at the local branch of the State University of New York.

My decision to leave teaching and pursue a doctorate was a practical one. I was struggling to support my family of three on a moderate four-figure teacher's income. One of my star chemistry students went to work for Eastman Kodak in Rochester, and she came back to Canton and took me out to dinner on her expense account. After that, I looked at myself in the mirror and said "What's wrong with this picture?" I then went to Temple University where I received my Doctor of Podiatric Medicine (DPM) degree in 1977. I was fortunate to be awarded an Army Health Professions Scholarship that paid my way for my four years in podiatry school at Temple. I then served four years as an Active-Duty Army podiatrist at Ft. Meade, Maryland.

After my Army service, I lived and practiced podiatry in politically correct Ithaca, New York from 1982-2001. During the time I practiced in Ithaca, I received an unusual form from the New York State Tax Department. It was entitled, "An Application for a Permit to Pay Employees by Check." I was instructed to fill out the form and mail it back to Albany with a check for twenty-five dollars. I immediately phoned my accountant who advised me to send in the form along with the check. It seems that the cash-strapped state at that time was looking for revenue sources wherever it could find them. My accountant explained the origin of this archaic regulation.

The stock market crash of 1929 occurred on Wall Street, NY, NY. Payroll checks from affected businesses bounced, and employees demanded their pay in cash. The State passed a law to certify that checks from businesses to pay employees henceforth must be valid. After the economic recovery, this outdated law remained on the books, but was overlooked until some Albany bean counter rediscovered it. The new enforcement of the old law was applied randomly, and my business was one of those selected. I joked with my employees about the new permit. I wish I still had a copy of it. I would frame it as an extreme example of government desperation and harassment.

One of the myriad things a doctor has to address upon opening a new practice is to obtain a DEA number. This allows him/her to write prescriptions for controlled substances such as narcotic pain medication. After leaving the Army and establishing my practice in Ithaca, I applied for my number. The Drug Enforcement Agency sent me my DEA number addressed to: "Evan F. Meltzer, DVM."

So, there it was; I could write prescriptions for furry patients but not for my human ones. This was somewhat ironic because Ithaca is home to Cornell University's Veterinary College. I actually had to contact my U. S. Senator's office to get the DVM changed to my correct degree designation, DPM.

Again, I wish I had saved that document.

In 2001, I sold my practice to a young doctor fresh out of his residency training who was carrying a six-figure school debt. He did not qualify for the amount of the loan required to buy the practice, and I was mandated by the Small Business Administration to hold a personal note for one-hundred-thousand dollars. The SBA structured the note such that sixty-five-thousand dollars was payable monthly over ten years at nine percent simple interest beginning immediately. The remaining thirty-five-thousand dollars was due in the year 2021, but accrued simple interest of nine percent until maturity. There was no requirement for partial payments on that portion of the loan.

In order to qualify for the huge loan to purchase the practice and the condominium unit my office was located in, he had to come up with a thirty-five-thousand dollar down payment. He had no money of his own, and his parents were either unwilling or unable to loan him the money. Time was growing desperately short and we needed to close the deal.

Along came the Good Fairy.

Linda liquidated some of her stocks to loan him the down payment and we had to pay the income tax on the net gains. In a separate deal between Linda and him, he agreed to pay off that loan from her soonest. Fortunately, he did so within a few months, with no interest payment to Linda.

Our buyer was keenly aware of the high interest rate of nine percent and its cumulative effect on the final value of the payoff amount. He was motivated to pay off the loan as soon as possible, but could not yet obtain commercial credit at a better interest rate until he proved to a conservative bank that he could successfully run my former successful practice by himself.

The "Land of Taxes" demanded from me their portion of state tax for the full one-hundred-thousand dollars for the 2002 tax year. My New Mexico accountant had never encountered this before. He said, "Income tax means you first get the income, and then you pay the tax." He also said "New York was being very aggressive in this matter."

His advice was, "Evan, you'd better pay the tax at the rate I calculate, because New York will most likely calculate a higher figure."

So, there it was, I had to pay income tax on money I had not received, and with no guarantee I would ever collect the full amount in my lifetime. After receiving my tax payment, New York State did send me a letter stating that my tax debt to them was fully satisfied from the sale of my practice. An interesting question arose. If my buyer had defaulted on this loan, could I have applied to New York for a prorated tax refund? My accountant didn't think so.

As previously mentioned, Ithaca is home to Cornell University, a member of the prestigious Ivy League. I wanted to apply there for college, but my parents said they could not afford to pay for that high-priced education. Cornell is the largest employer in Ithaca, and Linda worked there for a short time. Linda also worked for Ezra Cornell, the great, great…grandson of the original founder of the University, Ezra Cornell. He had his own financial consulting firm in Ithaca. Mr. Cornell was born a Trustee of the University and fathered a son, whose name was, you guessed it, Ezra.

Cornell truly is an "Ivory Tower" institution, with many of the academic staff stuffy and full of themselves. I found many of their professors to be difficult patients. I had one patient who was a professor of English. When I gave him a copy of my postoperative instructions, he took out a red pen from his pocket and corrected it! And I thought I had already graduated from college!

I also had the distinct honor to treat Nobel Laureates. They were the best and nicest people to deal with. They had nothing to prove to anyone. One day a chemistry professor who was a Nobel Laureate came to my office as a patient. As I walked into the treatment room, he asked me, "Dr. Meltzer, didn't I have you as a student in one of my chemistry classes?" I replied, "No sir, I did not have that honor. I did not go to Cornell."

Another Nobel Laureate in Physics, who worked on the Manhattan Project, was also my patient. He sent me post cards from his European trips. I made house calls to his 100-year-old mother-in-law, even shoveling snow from her sidewalk to get to her door. Many years later when I visited Los Alamos, New Mexico and his picture was in a scrapbook they had in their museum.

Not all of my former patients were college professors or Nobel Laureates. Most of my patients were ordinary folks, such as farmers, custodial workers, school teachers and so forth. One morbidly obese elderly woman whom I saw regularly decided to start smoking to lose weight. She didn't live much longer after choosing that unhealthy habit instead of a diet.

Among my favorite patients were several veterinarians who were sub specializing to become veterinary ophthalmologists, orthopedic surgeons, cardiologists and dermatologists. I could speak their language and also learn about their fascinating sub-specialties.

Ithaca is also home to lesser-known Ithaca College. It is a private college well known for its music school and physical therapy program. David Muir is one of their better-known alumni.

The stereotypical Ithaca College student was typified by a patient who came to my office wearing his Gucci loafers, Rolex watch, North Face ski parka, and drove to the office in the latest model Land Rover. He was a nice kid from Long Island, and I asked him if he skied, referring to his parka. He said, "No, but I like the jacket for this climate."

As he left the office, I sat thinking, "This kid can only go downhill from here in terms of possessions. How can he top this life after his daddy stops paying the bills?"

Ironically, it was often more difficult to collect money for my services from these rich kids' parents. Cornell, which has a large endowment, subsidizes many of its poorer students.

Linda and I lived at 20 Cedar Lane in Ithaca from 1994-2001, until we moved to New Mexico. One next door neighbor was a daughter of Rod Serling, who was born in Syracuse, NY. After just moving in, Ms. Serling came over to welcome us as new neighbors. She said, "I baked you chocolate chip cookies, but we ate them."

I will never forget that comment. Do I hear a distant sound of the *Twilight Zone* theme? Like father like daughter? I had the privilege of seeing Rod Serling when he visited the University of Colorado at Boulder while I was a graduate student there. Mr. Serling also had two male Serling cousins who were counsellors at a summer camp I went to on Seneca Lake in the 1950s.

The other next-door neighbor was a snobby Cornell professor and his equally snobby pediatrician wife. Our neighbor one street over was Carl Sagan and his wife, Ann Druyan and young daughter. Ms. Druyan wrote the screen play to the movie, *Contact* starring Jodie Foster. The story was taken from her husband's novel of the same title. Dr. Sagan's daughter needed podiatric care, and Ms. Druyan brought young Ms. Sagan into the office.

Ann Druyan was an intense woman who was focusing on a manuscript while I was treating her daughter. I asked her, "What are you working on?"

She said, "I'm working on the manuscript for the upcoming movie, *Contact*."

I jokingly asked, "Do you need any extras for the movie?"

I saw the movie but did not have a part in it. Ms. Sagan did fine with her treatment. I had the distinct pleasure of hearing Dr. Sagan lecture at Cornell before his untimely death from leukemia.

I also treated Ann Druyan's parents. One day my business manager came to me and said, "Doc, what kind of car is that?"

I looked out the window to see her parents parking a Bentley in front of the office.

Most people think that doctors are rich. While I don't deny most of us made a good living, the Bentley owners had Medicare insurance. Medicare at that time set their reimbursements to participating doctors at a lower level than their regular fees. Thus, as a participating doctor in Medicare I accepted the eighty percent that Medicare allowed for their treatment in spite of their enormous wealth and obvious ability to pay my usual fees for their care.

I also served as the podiatric consultant to Cornell's Student Health Center for two years. I saw student patients there on a fee-for-service basis. Billing was not a problem because my bills were sent to the college Bursar's office. The University would then send me a lump sum check at the end of the semester. If the bills went unpaid, the student in arrears would not be allowed to graduate until they settled up.

At first, I enjoyed going there. The Cornell campus is one of the most beautiful college campuses in the country ("High above Cayuga's waters") and it was a break from my own office routine. I was given an ID that allowed me to park and use the library and health facilities. I also gave several lectures to the Health Center staff. Near final exam time, however, students often failed to keep their appointments. I was left waiting for no-show patients while I was paying overhead in my own office. Eventually this became a financial decision, and I found it unprofitable to continue in that position.

Our house on Cedar Lane was built in 1963, and was situated on five acres of land on the brow of a steep hill. The house and pool sat on about one-and-a-half acres, with the remainder of the forested land on the steep hillside below. We had a 180-degree commanding view of Cayuga Lake, from Stewart Park in Ithaca to the south to Taughannock Falls State Park to the north. The house had an outdoor pool that could boast the finest view from a pool anywhere in the area. During our first summer at the house, Linda commented, "This is such a beautiful view it's a shame we can't share it as a park for others."

During the seven years we lived there, there were cars that stopped in front of our house to take pictures of the view of the lake on several occasions. I did not welcome the invasion of our privacy and directed them to the state parks in the area.

Cornell University spent a great deal of money on heating and cooling its campus buildings. The University was investigating ways in which to save money, and came up with the idea called

Lake Source Cooling. This was to become a system of pipes laid at the bottom of Cayuga Lake and pumped up to the campus. The temperature at the lake's bottom remained constant throughout the year, and would serve to cool the campus in summer and heat it in winter. Our house sat above the lake, and we watched barges bring the pipe sections for completion of this project. We left Ithaca before completion, but it was interesting to observe the progress. I have not heard what Cornell's return on their investment has been regarding their utility bills.

Our favorite event of the season was July fourth.

At sunset, many who lived in homes and cottages along the lake shore lit flares at a given time. It was a spectacular display of red flares extending for at least five miles along the lake's west shore. We could also see the fireworks display from the comfort of our yard coming from Ithaca College.

But best of all was watching the dozens of boats anchored off Stewart Park lined up to watch the fireworks. After the grand finale, they would all turn around and head back to their respective docks with all the colorful marine lights flashing and glowing and horns blaring.

We also had a good view of the dormitory tower at Ithaca College from our kitchen windows. While the students were away for the holidays, the custodial staff would turn on the lights in the tower a few days before New Years Eve with that year's numbers outlined by selected room lights on in the dorm rooms. At the stroke of midnight on New Years, the lights would change to the New Year. It was exciting to see ninety-nine change to zero-zero on the Y2K New Years eve.

Our house was a multi-level wood frame structure with low ceilings and original equipment single pane aluminum framed windows across the entire west side facing the lake. It was a large house with 4,200 square feet including a glassed-in conservatory. It had five bathrooms, four full bedrooms, a study, dining room, living room, and a partial basement with hot tub and redwood sauna. The house also needed a lot of work.

The couple we bought the house from did virtually no maintenance on the house, and we almost canceled the purchase offer when our inspector reported his findings. Our persuasive realtor hired another inspector who convinced us the house was ok.

The first winter, snow came through the poorly sealed windows in the kitchen.

We had to have the leaking buried fuel oil tank dug up and replaced. Our inspector did not discover that massive defect or we would have definitely walked away from the deal.

We replaced all the windows and sliding glass doors with triple pane low-E glass. The crumbling slate floors and inside steps were replaced with solid maple and oak. One of the bathrooms was remodeled. We paved the large gravel driveway with street pavement quality macadam. The exterior of the house had not been painted in years, and we had that job completed. We did extensive landscaping work outside. We came close to remodeling the kitchen but sold the house before tackling that expensive project.

All told, we put well over one-hundred-thousand dollars of improvements into the house, but the view and location were priceless. I could walk to my office, all uphill. Driving took five minutes. We did break even on the house sale.

Cayuga Lake is one of several Finger Lakes in the central New York region. These lakes are deep, long and narrow. Cayuga Lake is the longest at forty-four miles, and about four miles wide at its widest point. Seneca Lake to the west is forty miles long and at over six hundred feet deep is the deepest. An old Iroquois legend (these Native Americans prefer to be called Haudenosaunee) tells the story of the lakes' formations.

The Great Spirit created the earth, water and sky, and He was pleased with His work. As a stamp of approval, He placed His hand on the earth below, creating these lakes.

The geologic explanation is that the lakes were formed after the last Ice Age. Canadian glaciers carved deep narrow valleys from north to south that then became lakes after the glaciers melted. The only other similar lake formations I am aware of in the US are located in the northwest corner of Glacier National Park in Montana.

When my daughter Wendy was young, she was often fixated on the literal meaning of words. When I explained to her why the Finger Lakes were named as such, she said, "Dad, why aren't they called the Toe Lakes?" She also called toes, "Foot fingers." Her dad, uncle, and grandfather were all podiatrists.

When Wendy was three years old, she met her great grandmother for the first time. I said, "Wendy, this is your great grandmother."

She said as she looked up at her, "What's so great about her?"

At five years old, I introduced my daughter to a new friend. I said, "This is my daughter Wendy."

Wendy replied, "I'm not Wendy, I'm Doris!"

Many years later, "Doris" and I were dining out one evening at a nice restaurant and I was quite hungry. As I was eating my meal quickly, she said, "Dad, we're dining, not scarfing."

While Wendy was in high school, I answered the phone one evening. "Hello, is Dee there?"

I replied, "You must have the wrong number." Wendy was standing right next to me and said, "Dad, it's for me".

I never knew whether "Dee" was short for "WenDY" or "Doris".

She also coined a unique term for the bohemian type women so common in Ithaca at the time. Their typical uniform consisted of a braless tank top, underneath a pair of farmer's denim coveralls with combat boots. The hair was long; on their heads, legs and under the arm pits.

She called them, "Earth Muffins."

I mentioned that Ithaca was a politically correct town. It is a liberal place much like other college towns around the country.

A grocery store chain named Wegmans was opening up a store in Ithaca. The Wegman family founded Wegmans in 1913 in my hometown of Rochester. I grew up with my mother shopping in that store, and was excited they were locating in Ithaca. Wegmans had been listed as one of the 100 best places to work, and was named the top grocery chain in the U.S. by Consumer Reports (May 2009). It was a well- deserved honor, and Linda and I miss shopping there to this day. They are only located in the northeast.

A politically correct radical group in Ithaca suggested the new store be properly named, "WegPERSON". How ridiculous.

My son Peter, or Pete as he prefers to be called now, was only seven years old when his mother and I separated. We had shared custody for several years until his mother moved to Denver.

Pete would spend alternate weekends with me, and we shared many good father-son times together. One day, I was withdrawing money out of an ATM machine. Pete said,

"Dad, can we get one of those machines for the house?"

On the weekends he stayed with his mother, she signed him up for a Tae Kwon Do martial arts class at my local health club. I took him there on alternate Saturdays, and she took him on the Saturdays of her weekend. The classes were taught by a Black Belt instructor, and were open to any club member regardless of age. Students progressed and were tested for the next level belt. A white belt was a beginner, followed by yellow, green, etc. up until black. I decided that as long as I was taking him to class, I might as well attend myself. Eight-year-old Pete earned his yellow belt, and his dad was only a white belt. He really enjoyed his new status over his dad, and I know it was good for his self-confidence.

His mother stopped taking him to class on her weekends, and he fell behind. I kept going, and finally earned my own yellow belt. Later that summer, we went to a weekend camp for the martial arts, and had a great time.

I enjoyed the sport very much, but I was sparring with guys my own size, and the risk and incidence of injury was high. I withdrew from class to avoid injury, but I carried some skills I learned from this martial art into other sports. A few of my classmates became my patients due to foot injuries.

Pete was born in Philadelphia at the Hospital of the University of Pennsylvania (HUP) during my last year of podiatry school. My brother-in-law, Dr. Morrie Gold was Chief Resident of Ob-Gyn there, but did not deliver him. HUP was not located in one of Philadelphia's best neighborhoods. When I went to the nursery to see my son, the nurse asked me, "Sir, which one is yours?"

Pete was the only white baby born on that day at HUP.

Pete was born with a "wind swept deformity" of his feet. This is a condition where one foot turns in, and the other turns out, due to his spending time in a transverse position in the uterus.

Fortunately, one of my podiatry professors was one of the pre-eminent teachers of Podopediatrics, who specialized in treating the foot problems of children. I took him to Dr. James Ganley's private office, and he showed me how to apply corrective plaster casts to Pete's legs and feet to correct the deformities.

We were often stopped in public places and asked about what happened to our son. After growing tired of the involved explanations to strangers, I finally decided on brevity,

"He had a bad ski accident."

Pete was only three months old.

As I was about to graduate and move to Fort Meade, Maryland for my Army career, I asked Dr. Ganley, "Who should I take my son to for follow-up in Maryland?"

He quickly replied, "You take care of him yourself, after all, I trained you."

Dr. Ganley was one of the giants in our field, and he was the inventor of the Ganley Splint, a pediatric night splint. Unfortunately, he died of leukemia before his time.

At the time, the recommended follow up for Pete's problem was to fit him with custom foot orthotics that was changed every time he grew two shoe sizes until maturity.

The current theory then was that without that treatment, he probably would have developed other foot problems as an adult.

When Pete was fourteen, one day he said, "Dad, do I still need orthotics?"

I put on my doctor hat and examined him carefully.

"Pete, it looks like you don't need them anymore. What do you think would have happened if you didn't have orthotics?" Pete quickly replied,

"I would have walked around in circles."

Soon after we moved into Cedar Lane, Linda began to suffer with some medical problems. Ithaca has a terrible winter climate and shares with other central New York communities (e.g. Syracuse) a reputation of having the least amount of sunshine per year of any area in the U.S., including Seattle. Cloudy conditions can last up to two weeks without seeing the sun once. The locals refer to a common combination of snow and freezing rain as, "It's Ithacating."

Summers and the fall foliage are usually beautiful as is the surrounding countryside.

One of Linda's diagnoses was "Seasonal Affective Disorder." This is a common condition in the northern U.S. climates and in Scandinavian countries. We purchased a special natural spectrum light that approximates sunlight to fight this disorder that Linda used for sewing and reading. Linda was afflicted with other medical problems, and we began a discussion of our eventual relocation to a place with a better climate. It is not a quick process to sell a private solo podiatry practice, and find employment in the same profession in a good climate. We had vacationed in Cancun, Costa Rica, Florida, Arizona, New Mexico, California, and Linda went to Antigua for a week to recover from surgery while I remained behind to work. We knew there were better climates around.

I applied for and received podiatry licenses in Florida and Arizona.

During the winter of 1998-1999, Linda rented a small place in Pompano Beach, Florida. My parents were renting a place nearby, and could stay in touch with her. I visited as often as I could. After living there for about six weeks, Linda was driving along a quiet street and was rear ended by a distracted sixteen-year-old girl in her daddy's Jeep. Linda suffered ruptured discs, a concussion and whiplash. We hired the wrong Florida lawyer and received no settlement from the other party.

The following winter, 1999-2000 we rented a place in Green Valley, Arizona. Fortunately, Linda's time there was uneventful, but we both learned to love the southwest. Again, I visited as often as I could while maintaining my Ithaca practice. We had driven through Albuquerque to and from Arizona and liked what we saw.

One of the highlights of my career occurred during this period. I had been seeking a position on the New York State Board for Podiatry for about five years. The Board consisted of a podiatrist from each part of the state and two non-professional citizen members. Finally, there was an opening in my part of the State, and I applied. I drove to Albany for a personal interview with the Executive Director. I was selected and appointed to the Board.

New York State had the largest number of practicing podiatrists of any state. The Board met quarterly in New York City. I would fly from Ithaca's Tompkins County Airport to JFK in New York, and then take a cab downtown for the Board meetings. I retraced my steps after the meeting, and would arrive home the same evening. I found my service as a board member very gratifying, and received a wonderful letter of appreciation from the Executive Director and a certificate from the President of the State University of New York thanking me for my service. I still have those letters.

Moving to New Mexico necessitated my resigning from the board before my term expired. After I drove Linda back to Ithaca from Green Valley in the spring of 2000, I began my job search in earnest. Of course, we had to stop at Taos Ski Valley in New Mexico on the way home so I could ski there for a day.

Medical malpractice is not well understood by the general public. The outrageous examples, such as leaving an instrument in a patient's belly or wrong site surgery as in amputating the wrong leg have been much publicized. There are safeguards now in place to minimize these events that will be explained in a further chapter. What the public does not realize is that few doctors actually malpractice. Most suits are brought about by patients who may be unhappy with a result of a medical treatment, or who had a billing dispute with the doctor's office, or were encouraged to sue by family, friends, or by lawyers' advertisements that promise, "you don't pay a legal fee unless we collect." Sometimes the careless comments of another doctor can trigger a lawsuit.

Every physician who practices in a hospital was required to carry a multi-million- dollar malpractice insurance policy at his or her considerable expense. Most insurers offer discounts to its members who participate in risk management programs. These are either home study programs or formal lecture sessions given at major medical meetings. They are intended to educate the physician on ways to reduce their risk of being sued. This includes instructions on proper medical documentation, doctor-patient interpersonal relationships, and a host of other factors that lessen the risk.

Doctors are human and sometimes make mistakes. Several states are now allowing doctors to admit medical errors to their patients without risk of legal retaliation. Other states like Texas had limits of $250,000 on malpractice awards, much to the consternation of Texas malpractice attorneys.

It is generally accepted among physicians in private practice that if you practice long enough, it's not a matter of "if" you will get sued; it's a matter of "when". The public also does not realize that being sued for malpractice is a life changing event for the defendant doctor, regardless of the eventual outcome. Once a doctor suspects or actually is notified of a pending action, he/she should immediately contact their malpractice insurance carrier. In most cases, after reviewing the relevant details, the insurance company will recommend that the doctor settle out of court for a negotiated amount. The advantage of a negotiated settlement is that a trial is avoided. Malpractice trials are expensive and the outcomes are uncertain, regardless of the strength of the defendant doctor's case. There are so many variables, including jury makeup, the skill of the opposing lawyers, the quality of the expert witnesses and the judge's bias. True justice does not always prevail.

The downside to settling a claim is that this is reported directly to the National Practitioner Data Bank. Both civilian and government hospitals and other related organizations have access to this information, and will always include a search of the Data Bank as part of a background check during the credentialing process for a doctor applying for hospital privileges or a job. Most hospitals understand the problem of nuisance suits, and will often overlook small settlements after appropriate investigation and reviewing that doctor's explanation of the incident.

Every application for hospital privileges or for a government health care provider job includes a question similar to the one below.

On VA Form 10-2850, the application for a job at the VA for physicians, dentists, podiatrists and optometrists, Item #33 on page 3 of the application asks:

> "ARE YOU NOW, OR HAVE YOU EVER BEEN, INVOLVED IN ADMINISTRATIVE, PROFESSIONAL OR JUDICIAL PROCEEDINGS IN WHICH MALPRACTICE ON YOUR PART IS OR WAS ALLEGED? "(If "yes" give details including name of action or proceedings, date filed, court or reviewing agency, and the status or

disposition of case concerning allegations, together with your explanation of the circumstances involved.) As a provider of health care services, the VA has an obligation to exercise reasonable care in determining that applicants are properly qualified. It is recognized that many allegations of professional malpractice are proven groundless. Any conclusion concerning your answer as it relates to professional qualifications will be made only after a full evaluation of the circumstances involved.)"

In summary, if a doctor is ever sued, the answer to that question must always be "yes". If there is an out of court settlement or jury award to the plaintiff patient, it is reported to the National Practitioner Data Bank. The best outcome for a defendant doctor is for a jury to announce a not guilty verdict, but the answer to the above question must always be "yes." There is no reporting to the Data Bank for a verdict in favor of the defendant doctor.

In 1995, Dr. Berman, a family physician practicing in Ithaca and also my distant cousin, referred me a patient who had stepped on a toothpick. He attempted to remove it in his office without success, and sent her to me. I informed the patient that I would also attempt a removal in the office, but if that were not successful, I would have to take her to the hospital operating room. She agreed and consented in writing to this treatment plan. Up to this point in my career, my success rate for removing foreign bodies from the foot was one hundred percent. I felt confident I would be able to do this. The problem with wooden objects is that they do not show up on standard x-rays. Furthermore, this woman had been walking on her injured foot for some time before coming to my office. In all likelihood, the toothpick had moved.

I was not successful removing the toothpick in the office under local anesthesia. About two weeks later, I took her to the operating room. After spending about an hour surgically exploring for the alleged toothpick, I made the decision that I might cause more harm by continuing my search, and I stopped. At that point, I was not even certain the toothpick was still there.

I placed the woman on crutches and antibiotics, and told her that if the toothpick were still in her foot, we would know it after she completed the course of antibiotics. It would fester. She was also instructed not to walk on the foot for fear of it migrating.

Mr. Murphy's Law prevailed, and sure enough, her foot developed an abscess. I consulted one of our local radiologists for advice on the best imaging test to positively identify the location of the toothpick, and she recommended an MRI. This was a twelve-hundred-dollar test, and the patient's insurance had lapsed. The next best test, according to the radiologist was a CT scan. This was a less expensive test, and the patient consented to it. Sure enough, the CT scan revealed the presence of the toothpick. It had migrated from the bottom of her foot almost to the top surface. I asked my good friend and former brother-in-law podiatrist from Cortland if he would assist me in the surgery. He agreed.

It took both of us experienced Board-Certified foot surgeons two hours to finally locate and remove the toothpick.

Postoperatively, the patient did fine and recovered uneventfully. Unfortunately for me, she owed me quite a bit of money for all the services I had provided. She knew prior to her initial visit with me that her insurance had run out. She kept misleading me into believing she was covered by having my office check her coverage with various companies well into her treatment until it was clear to me she had no coverage. Her husband was an acquaintance, and I called him myself one day. "Larry, your wife has an outstanding bill of fourteen-hundred dollars for all my work."

He said, "Well, it had to come out anyway."

I replied, "Yes it did, but I do not work for free."

He said, "Can we work out a payment plan?"

I did not have a good experience with patient payment plans. Most people will pay for a few months, and then conveniently forget the balance necessitating collection proceedings for the balance due.

I asked, "What did you have in mind?"

He replied, "How about fourteen dollars per month?"

I quickly did the math. "Larry, that will take one hundred months, and that's not acceptable."

We ended the conversation on that note.

I gave much thought about what to do about this situation. I had provided good and ultimately successful service to the patient in good faith, while they knew all along that they had no insurance. The more I thought about it, the angrier I became. This was clearly theft of service. After consulting an attorney, I decided to file suit for the money owed. If you ask most doctors, they will advise not to do this because it can result in a counter suit for malpractice. That was exactly what happened. Before I go into the details, do you believe I was guilty of malpractice?

About a month after I filed suit to collect my professional fees, I was served papers alleging malpractice. I immediately contacted my insurance company who assigned me an attorney from a law firm in Syracuse, New York. The plaintiff's attorney was a relative of theirs who practiced in their nearby city of Cortland. My daughter was born in Cortland, and my former in-laws lived and practiced podiatry in that small community for over fifty years.

My assigned attorney, Nate Ward was young, but had tried several medical malpractice cases before. I had no choice in attorney selection because my insurance company was paying his fees. I had to rely that my insurer would retain a good attorney to protect our mutual interests. I had done some legal defense work for the same Syracuse law firm of Mr. Ward as an expert witness for other defendant podiatrists insured by my same company. I was asked on several occasions to be a plaintiff witness by other law firms. Before this action against me, I always lived by the motto, "But for the Grace of God could go me." I never had, and never would have testified against one of my colleagues, although the money was good for doing so.

My memory of the legal proceedings between 1995 and 2000 was cloudy, but I recall that my insurance company initially recommended I settle this as a nuisance suit. I refused, since I knew I did not malpractice. Negotiations dragged on, and depositions were taken from the plaintiff and me. Nate Ward was not sure he could win this case when the plaintiff suddenly hired another lawyer. Their relative attorney was clearly out of his league, since medical malpractice is a legal specialty requiring sophisticated knowledge of medicine. Apparently, the home town relative lawyer was owed a big favor, and somehow managed to get his client's case represented by the nastiest malpractice attorney in Syracuse.

During this time, my wife, Linda was my trusted office manager. My income rose significantly with her managing the financial aspect of the practice. She steadfastly refused to let me settle this case, as she was as angry as I was that these people could maliciously use the legal system to avoid payment of a medical bill.

If the case were decided in their behalf, either by trial or settlement, they stood to make money at my expense.

In order for our marriage to work, Linda and I agreed to not discuss business matters after work. The problem was we would often work in the office on weekends to catch up on paperwork. By 1999, the stress of managing a medical office (and maybe by having me as her daytime "boss") brought on a severe case of fibromyalgia. Linda had to retire. Of course, she had intimate knowledge of all aspects of the legal case against me.

The financial stakes were getting higher with negotiations between the attorneys, and at Linda's urging; I finally decided to go to trial. The contract I signed with my malpractice insurance company allowed me the final say in this matter, and they were obligated to pay for my costs related to a trial. I reasoned that I was in the process of looking for a job as an employed podiatrist. I did not wish to have a blemish on my record that might jeopardize a new position, so I decided to leave my fate up to a jury of my peers.

On the Tuesday after Labor Day in 2000, jury selection began. In New York, a trial like this one required only six jurors. The only caveat was that their decision must be unanimous. During the proceedings, Linda sat in the observer's section of the Cortland County Courthouse sewing patches for a quilt. She kept a keen eye on the reactions of the jurors during the examination and cross examination process.

My insurance company hired a podiatrist from Syracuse who served as my expert witness. We did not know each other, and I had no input regarding his selection. He did an adequate job of defending me. I was a well- known podiatrist throughout New York State. I had been President of the Southern Tier Division of the New York State Podiatric Medical Association, and as previously mentioned was appointed as a member of the State

Board for Podiatry. While establishing my practice in Ithaca, I practiced part-time in Cortland with my former in-laws.

Because of my good state-wide reputation, the plaintiff could not find another podiatrist in the entire state of New York who would agree to testify as an expert witness against me. They finally found a "hired gun" from Philadelphia, PA. I recognized his name but did not know him personally, as I had completed my podiatry studies in Philadelphia. He spent about equal time practicing podiatry as he did testifying against his colleagues. Nate Ward was not as well prepared as his adversary, but he was quick on his feet. When he asked the plaintiff's expert, "Did you know that Dr. Meltzer was on the Board of Podiatry for New York?"

The expert answered, "I'm sorry to hear that."

The local jury did not like that response. I felt betrayed. How could a supposed colleague who did not even know me personally react like that? I felt like bolting out of my seat and hurting him. Money may really be the root of all evil.

Nate destroyed him on cross examination.

Dr. Berman and the radiologist were also called to testify. Linda continued to work patiently on her quilt, and quietly observe the jury.

In a surprise move, the Plaintiff's attorney called Linda to the stand. This was completely unexpected by everyone. Nate Ward's relative inexperience failed to prepare us for this possibility. Most witnesses are prepared before they are called to the stand, but Linda was not afforded that opportunity. She did very well under the circumstances, recalling what she could and answering truthfully. I could see that the jury felt sorry for her.

One rule Nate drilled into me in preparation for the trial was that I should never vary from my sworn deposition taken about two years before. I prepared for my trial like I was studying for a final exam in college; reviewing the plaintiff's depositions and mine.

Nate was a master at cross examining the plaintiff, and exposed glaring errors in her current testimony compared to her earlier deposition. The jury took notice.

Finally, on Friday, the fourth day of the trial, the judge ordered the jury to deliberate.

They were gone for not more than an hour when the foreman was ready to announce the verdict.

The judge asked, "How do you find the defendant?"

The foreman replied, "We find the defendant not guilty."

The plaintiff was ordered to pay all court costs and my original bill.

She did not appeal.

As I thanked the members of the jury outside the court room, one of the jurors told me, "There are too many lawsuits, and we don't like to see our good doctors get sued."

That was good enough for me. My insurance company paid me a token sum for my time away from my office, and promptly raised my premiums.

Linda completed the quilt. At my request, she stitched the word, "VERITAS" above her name on the back of the quilt.

"The truth shall set you free."

***

A few steps below the fear of a malpractice case is the worry of an audit by Medicare.

Medicare is the government subsidized health care insurance program for retired and disabled individuals as I had previously described. Many older people suffer from foot problems and thus many of my patients had Medicare as their primary insurance plan.

Unlike private insurance companies who can simply drop you from their preferred provider list, Medicare fraud is a federal offense, punishable by fines, imprisonment, or both. One of the worst nightmares experienced by doctors in private practice is the dreaded Medicare audit. This is a process where Medicare contacts a particular provider announcing that they are coming to the office to review patient charts. They instruct the provider to cancel all patient appointments for that day, and be ready to present requested patient charts upon their arrival. They will not give you the names in advance.

The formal closing of the sale of my Ithaca practice took place on July first. I was planning to leave for New Mexico in a month, and I spent the time in my office with the new doctor who purchased my practice introducing him to his soon-to-be patients.

In the middle of July, I received a call from Medicare that they were scheduling an audit of my practice. They were unaware I had sold the practice, and the new doctor and I wanted to keep it that way. Any problems Medicare might uncover were mine anyway.

The dreaded day came, and the new doctor disappeared for the day per our mutual arrangement. Three officials from the local Medicare office showed up carrying their own copier. They slapped a list of twenty names on my reception desk and requested to review those patient's charts. Their demeanor was professional, and I treated them with deference and respect. My staff and I made sure their needs were met. The group spent the day in my office conference room reviewing and copying pertinent parts of the charts, and left that afternoon. Meanwhile, I could not treat patients while they were in my office in case they had questions. This cost the new doctor and me a day of lost income.

I was told I would not hear back from them for "some time."

* * *

One of the requirements of having a medical license is that you must keep current in your field. All states have various requirements for continuing medical education credits (CME) for license renewal. I've been licensed to practice in seven states and the District of Columbia, so I am quite familiar with these regulations.

In November 1993, Linda and I travelled to Costa Rica for a CME meeting. It was held at a beautiful resort on the Pacific coast. The CME lectures were held in the early mornings, and there was ample time to sight see or relax in the afternoons.

We extended our trip to further explore Costa Rica after the conclusion of the meeting, with an ad-on trip to Guatemala.

Our travel agency provided us with a personal guide to take us around the sights in Guatemala. The itinerary for the last day of our trip was to take us to the famous Mayan site of Tikal. We planned to leave the country the next day.

Tikal is in a remote part of Guatemala. Back then, in order to get there, we flew from Guatemala City to a jungle airstrip in the central part of the country. From there, we took a bus for two hours to the entrance to the Mayan ruins. We were with a group of other tourists including Canadians who worked for United Airlines. Our group met with a local Tikal guide who proceeded to take us on a one hour trek through the ruins.

It had rained the night before. The jungle was wet and the rocks were slippery. I was busy taking pictures and fell behind the group. As I hurried to catch up with the group, I slipped on a wet mossy rock. I heard a crack and pop, and saw my right foot externally rotated from my right knee. In lay terms, if my right knee was at 12-o'clock, my right foot was facing 3- o'clock.

Since I am a podiatrist, I knew exactly what had happened to me. I had just suffered one of the worst ankle fractures you can get.

The pain had not yet broken through my shock, and I lay on my back looking up through my sunglasses at the brilliant sky above, listening to and watching the howler monkeys screech as they swung through the jungle canopy above.

My first thoughts were, "How am I ever going to get out of this place?"

My next thoughts were, "What's going to happen to my practice, and who's going to do my surgery?" I knew I needed surgery.

By the time I started feeling pain, Linda's worried face appeared above me.

She asked, "What happened?"

As I explained, I began to examine my leg to see if there was an open fracture with exposed bone. Fortunately, my self-examination was negative for an open fracture, but I realized I could not take even one step on my broken ankle, or the bone could become exposed thus creating a much more serious open fracture.

An old Army phrase came to mind, "We were in deep kimchee."

Linda summoned the guide and told him to go get help. They gently placed me into the back of a pickup truck and I held my leg as steady as I could over the very bumpy trail.

At that point, the pain was really taking over.

Codeine was then available over the counter in Canada without a prescription. My new Canadian friends found some pills, and I gladly took them. We were expected to get back to the jungle airport in a few hours to retrace our trip back to Guatemala City. I also knew there was no way I was going to have any medical care in that third world country.

They took me into the filthy town outside of Tikal for medical help. I knew I was the most qualified professional in the area to treat this injury, but I was the patient!

I asked Linda to try to get us to the equivalent of a drug store so she could purchase some ibuprofen and some plaster for casting my leg.

As I was lying on my back in the back seat of a van with my twisted foot hanging out of the door, a local came up to me and said, "Señor, I fix your foot for you."

I screamed, "Get away from me!"

I was able to observe and smell the raw sewage running along the street next to the van.

By the time I scared away the local witch doctor, Linda arrived with the medication and the plaster. I knew that a closed reduction of my fracture was not possible and that surgery was inevitable. I also knew I had to immobilize my injury in its current position until I arrived back in the U.S. for definitive care.

I instructed Linda on how to apply the plaster casting rolls, knowing full well that sometime in the next few hours that swelling would be a real problem. We would have to eventually figure out a way to bi-valve (split open) the hard cast. In developed countries, this is accomplished with a specialized cast cutting saw. I had one in my Ithaca office.

I popped the ibuprofen pills to help control the pain and swelling, and arrived at the jungle airstrip with a hard cast over my deformed foot and leg. I had no crutches, and was helped aboard the plane by my new friends. Some big shot from the local government was also a passenger, so he got preferred seating in spite of my obvious pain and injury.

We finally landed at the Guatemala City airport. We were due to fly out of there the next day.

We had several problems.

Our passports and all our belongings were in our hotel away from the airport. My foot and leg were beginning to swell, and my pain was becoming unbearable. The airport closed at 6 pm, and was under armed guard by soldiers wielding sub-machine guns. Our scheduled flight was not due to depart until the following afternoon.

Linda tried to hire a private jet to get us to Miami, the nearest U.S city.

Her Spanish was rudimentary and mine nonexistent. After considerable back and forth negotiations, we were able to find a plane and pilot who would fly us to Miami for nine thousand dollars. His main problem was filing a flight plan and getting that approved by a corrupt government on a Saturday evening. I also made two telephone calls.

One was to my good friend and tropical medicine specialist, Dr. Jerry H in Ithaca.

After reaching him and consulting with him, we both agreed that as long as I had palpable pulses in my foot, I should get the hell out of there as soon as possible.

My other call was to the American Embassy.

There was no answer.

After my recovery, I sent then-Secretary of State Warren Christopher a scathing letter. I received an unsatisfactory reply from an undersecretary.

My new Canadian airline friends managed to book us on the next redeye leaving at 3am to Miami.

During this time, I sat on the tarmac with my leg hanging out of the van door and the airport had closed for the night. The armed soldiers stood over us. We managed to talk our way out of that tense situation so we could return to our hotel.

The people in our tour group left before us, and packed up our luggage in our room. However, we had to return to the hotel because our passports were in the hotel's safe.

My toes were turning purple and the pain was unbearable due to the swelling. After a long time, Linda got a pair of rusty scissors from a hotel maid, and she somehow was able to split the cast. It took her almost two hours, but my pain relief was immediate.

Jimmy Buffett wrote a song entitled, *Everyone Has a Cousin in Miami,* It's on his "Fruitcakes" album. I am no exception.

I called my cousin Howard in Miami, who agreed to meet us the next morning at the airport and to hook me up with a good orthopedic surgeon.

The red-eye flight had few passengers and I was able to lie across a row of seats. Linda kept applying ice packs on my split cast throughout the several hour flight. A week later would have been Thanksgiving week, and we might not have been so fortunate as to get a flight at the last minute.

Howard met us at 6 am in Miami, and drove us to the hospital. I checked into the emergency department, my cast was removed and I finally had x-rays. I also got a shot of Demerol for my pain.

I asked the x-ray tech if I could see my films. He said, "No, I can't show them to you, but I'm glad it's not my ankle."

The ER doctor on duty allowed me to review my x-rays. I had a pronation-external rotation fracture of my right ankle. In non-medical terms, my ankle was a mess.

The doctor said, "It is standard protocol to sedate you and attempt a closed reduction of your fracture."

I said, "Doc, you and I both know the only way to fix this is with surgery. I'll wait for the orthopedist."

Howard's orthopedist was on the golf course that morning, but he finally arrived at 10 am. After reviewing the x-rays, he gave me two options: He could recast me and send me back to Ithaca for surgery, or he could perform the surgery here.

I said, "Doc, do it here." He grinned from ear to ear. His reaction was almost like a small child who says,

"Oh, can I really."

That's my kind of surgeon.

In addition to his enthusiasm, he was the team orthopedist for the University of Miami sports teams, which was good enough for me.

After the surgery was finished and on the way to the recovery room, I asked in my drug-fogged state, "Doc, how long did the surgery take?" He said, "Five hours."

I replied, "Five hours, what took you so long?"

My heart monitor stopped as I was being wheeled to recovery. I shouted, "I'm DEAD."

"Better living through chemistry."

I stayed four days in that hospital. I left with a Miami Heat fiberglass cast on my leg. I wanted a Miami Dolphins cast, but one of the other orthopedists' sons broke his arm that weekend and got the last Dolphins cast. Linda arranged for the practice to have coverage until my return by my former brother-in-law and still close friend from Cortland.

I stayed at cousin Judi's house in Boca Raton for another week until my first postoperative visit and then flew back to Ithaca.

Due to the nature of the surgery, I still had one remaining screw in my ankle that would eventually require surgical removal. I was not allowed to bear any weight on my right leg for three months due to the risk of breaking the screw. During that time, I could not drive. Linda drove me to the office every day, and I treated patients from a wheelchair. Swelling was a real problem. I would see one patient and then I had to elevate my leg for 15 minutes before I could see another patient.

After two months, my cast was removed but I was still not permitted to walk without crutches. One screw had to be removed first; otherwise walking on the ankle could break the screw. By now, it was in the dead of winter in Upstate New York. I could drive, but I still needed to use crutches. One day driving home from the office in my Toyota Camry station wagon, I got stuck in the snow at the bottom of the hill. I got out of the car, grabbed my crutches and slogged (I don't think you can trudge using crutches) uphill through foot deep snow the one-quarter mile to my house. When I arrived home, I announced to Linda, "Tomorrow I'm going shopping for a four-wheel drive vehicle."

The very next day I drove to the local Toyota dealer, and traded in my wagon for a used Toyota 4Runner. It was previously owned by a friend of mine who worked at the dealership, so I knew it was in good shape. I never had to slog or trudge for the rest of that winter.

My income was affected during that three-month period. My hospital allowed me to perform surgery on my patients from my wheelchair. Everyone was very understanding. Finally, it was time for my second operation to remove the screw that was keeping me from walking.

The OR schedule on that day was interesting.

I was listed as the surgeon for two cases, and then I was listed as a patient of my local orthopedist on the same schedule. I remember finishing my cases, then climbing onto the operating table in my scrubs to have my screw removed under local anesthesia.

Sometime after my recovery, Linda said, "Evan, if I ever get the urge to visit another country, I'm going shopping at Pier One Imports and eating at a Chinese restaurant."

I am convinced that if it were not for my wife's heroic actions, my bleached bones would be resting in the Guatemala jungle to this day.

* * *

I applied for a position at the VA in Albuquerque. I was sent a list of questions to answer via email. Sometime after submitting my answers, I received a call from the senior podiatry resident in Albuquerque who said she was asked to call me by her chief, whom I shall call IS (stands for insecure schmuck). That call culminated in an offer for a fully funded job interview. I was expected to deliver a lecture to the residents and staff podiatrists.

In September, after the trial, Linda and I flew to Albuquerque and were put up at the upscale Westin Hotel, near the Albuquerque Sunport. I was to be picked up the next morning by one of the residents. That evening we enjoyed complementary cocktails and refreshments on the penthouse level, while watching pairs of F-16 fighter planes taking off from nearby Kirtland Air Force Base. So far so good.

My ride was late picking me up the next morning. He got into a fender-bender accident in heavy morning traffic, but was unhurt. We arrived at the VA about 9 am. My lecture was scheduled for lunch hour after clinic. I was dressed in a suit, and the resident who picked me up introduced me to the others. IS was nowhere in sight. The residents and students began to bombard me with clinical questions, as they saw as many as forty-five patients per morning. I gladly rolled up my sleeves and helped them out. I later found out it was the right thing to do. Other candidates for the job were reluctant to help the residents during their interviews.

Finally, IS strolled in about 10:30 am, having been to a doctor's appointment. He was thrown from his horse and broke his arm, but was nearing the end of his treatment.

We finished clinic and headed for lunch with sandwiches provided, and I gave my lecture. Also present was a civilian podiatrist from the community who would pitch in when IS was away.

There was a surgical case scheduled for that afternoon, and I was invited to observe. I gave my suggestions. I was tested all day, in clinic with being asked to interpret x-rays, in my lecture, and in surgery.

After surgery, IS invited me to talk with him in his office. After a long discussion, he offered me the job.

The resident drove me back to the hotel where I could tell Linda the news. I remember riding in his truck overwhelmed with emotion. This was the beginning of a new chapter of "My Interesting Life."

I found Linda at the hotel pool, and told her the good news. Linda likes to plan ahead as much as possible, and her first thoughts were of housing.

The plan that evening was for IS and his wife, Linda and me, and the civilian podiatrist and his wife to drive to Santa Fe for dinner. We ate at one of the finest places in town, and it was IS's treat. The other doctor offered to contribute, but IS said this was partial payment for his volunteering in the clinic. Upon parting company, I told IS, "I have to sell my practice and my house, so don't expect me anytime soon."

He responded, "I know that. I've been working alone for over eight years, so I can wait a little longer until you are ready."

Upon arriving back in Ithaca, we told no one about my job offer. I knew that the value of a practice is upheld by the reputation of its owner, and telling my patients too soon might cause them to leave my practice and seek care elsewhere.

I finally received my formal letter of hire from my-soon-to-be new boss who was also IS's boss; the Chief of Surgical Service at the Albuquerque VA. Once I received that official letter, I could formally begin looking for a buyer and we could list our house for sale. I don't recall what reason we gave our friends for selling our house. Maybe it was to downsize due to Linda's health.

I listed my practice for sale with a practice broker. He was able to locate my eventual buyer who grew up near Rochester and wanted to practice near his hometown. In February, he and his wife flew in from Chicago where he was completing his residency, and Linda and I took them out to dinner. They were impressed with the office and dinner, and we began negotiations through the practice broker.

My podiatry office was my third office location in Ithaca since my arrival in 1982. The Village Office Campus, built in 1988 was a cluster of condominium buildings occupied by various medical specialists, dentists, a large real estate office, and others. I purchased my 2100 square foot condominium from an insurance company in 1994. The space was professionally remodeled into a podiatry office, with Linda acting as the interior decorator. It also had a 2100 square foot basement, plenty of free parking, and was located across the street from the major shopping mall in Ithaca. It was truly a beautiful and functional office in a prime location, and my buyer and his wife were sold.

The broker warned me not to tell any of my patients of the impending sale and for me to maintain my productivity and hence the practice's value. Through the extensive documents I sent him including a complete inventory down to the last Band-Aid; accounting records and copies of tax returns, he set the sale price for my practice. Both my buyer and I agreed on his valuation. Selling a medical practice is as much art as science, with many types of formulas in use. My broker based the sale on as much fixed assets as he could to protect both parties. Linda and I found it difficult to not discuss our future plans with our Ithaca friends. Both of our families lived out of town so we could talk with them.

Linda and I flew to Albuquerque on a house-hunting trip in April.

Chapter 2

NEW MEXICO,

Land of Enchantment
2001-2004

We awoke in our empty home of seven years on Cedar Lane in Ithaca, New York for the final time on the last day of July, 2001. We drove to our lawyer's office for the closing on the house, but we left the door to the conservatory of our home unlocked so we could return afterwards to let the dogs run in their yard for the last time before driving to New Mexico.

As we got out of the car from downtown Ithaca, I said to Linda, "I'm going to really miss this beautiful view of the lake." She replied, "We'll be replacing this view with a different one in New Mexico. We'll have a great view of Sandia Mountains."

She also said, "Evan, I think I now know what my purpose in life really is."

"What is it?"

"I'm looking over my beautiful landscaping we worked on for the last seven years, and I think I'm meant to beautify this earth one property at a time."

Little did either of us realize at the time she would get several more chances in the next few years. I said, "We'll have to learn a whole new way of gardening in the arid southwest."

It was a typical beautiful summer day, reminding me of the day I visited Ithaca before leaving the Army. I sat with my then brother-in-law on the Ithaca Commons observing the vibrant shops and foot traffic, and decided at that moment I would establish my practice there.

Linda and I, along with our dogs Sparky, Lucky, Muffin and Precious loaded into the Mountaineer SUV for our next great adventure.

Columbus, Ohio is a full day's drive from Ithaca, and that's where both of my children lived. We spent that night at my son Pete's house. Actually, it was still Pete's wife's parents 'home at that time. The closing on our new home in Bernalillo, New Mexico was done via fax and phone, so we took possession of the house upon our arrival there. I remember that it was raining as we pulled into the garage of our new home. Fortunately, I delayed my start at the VA until late August to give us time to settle into the new environment.

We left Ithaca without a dime in our pockets from the sale of my practice. That closing was delayed for several weeks due to the bureaucracy of dealing with the Small Business Administration and attorneys. I was forced to hold a note for a hundred-thousand-dollars with the balance of the sale funded by an agency of the SBA. As described in the New York Chapter, I had no choice in this matter, and would have much preferred to get the hundred-thousand-dollars at the time of sale. The young doctor who purchased my practice was so stretched financially that he could not afford to purchase my accounts receivable. I had to make arrangements with my former business manager to work these accounts. He felt guilty about leaving my employ to work for the local neurosurgeon, so he agreed to work my accounts after his regular hours at the neurosurgeon's office. The new doctor allowed my former manager office and computer access for him to do my work. It turns out I ended up collecting only pennies on the dollar while paying him well to work the accounts for about nine months. The neurosurgeon lost his surgical privileges at Cayuga Medical Center, the hospital in Ithaca where I also performed surgery, and my old manager subsequently lost his job as his new employer closed his practice.

We spent the time before my VA start date to find the Bernalillo Post Office, get New Mexico drivers and car licenses, and to shop for the new house. I spent some of this time building a work bench and storage cabinets for the garage from kits. DWI was such a problem in New Mexico that in 2001 all drivers under the age of forty were required to take a mandatory course on the subject. Linda and I were exempt from the course due to our tender ages.

I arrived at the VA on a Monday in late August, dressed in a coat and tie. It was the last day I wore a tie to work until my final day a year-and-a half later. My first stop was to the podiatry clinic, where I was promptly descended upon by residents hungry for knowledge. The Chief of Podiatry, who I will still refer to as IS (insecure schmuck) had not yet shown up for the morning clinic, and the residents were eager for guidance. One of these residents approached me with a patient presentation, and said, "Will you review these x-rays with me?"

"I haven't even been to the HR Department yet so I can get paid." I replied.

I answered his questions and then quickly walked over to Human Resources. I spent the better part of my first week going through the standard new employee orientation programs and signing up for the various government benefits available.

One highlight of that week was learning about the Navajo Code Talkers of World War II, several of whom resided in New Mexico, which is one of the three states that encompasses the Navajo Nation.

By the following week, I was ready to devote my full efforts to the residents and patients. The standard duty hours for a Title 38 VA employee (doctor) were 8-4:30. I usually arrived at my office at about 7:30 am and got to clinic by 8 am. I soon learned that "Chief", the residents' nickname for IS, rarely arrived in clinic before 10:30 am. I was the only on-site attending doctor from eight until IS wandered into clinic. The podiatric residency had been running like that for years until I arrived. The residents and students were the cream of the crop, but I uncovered some serious errors in their treatment of patients due to lack of oversight from IS.

I discovered nothing life-threatening, but in my opinion patient safety was compromised due to lack of proper supervision. The VA educational system nationwide had been severely criticized for this problem, and if what I saw in Albuquerque was the tip of the iceberg, the VA had a big problem. Since that time, all medical specialties who train and supervise residents in the Veterans Health Administration have become much more responsible with specific written policies implemented and enforced by Washington. A local civilian podiatrist occasionally volunteered to supervise the clinic before my arrival when IS took a vacation or attended a meeting.

There was a massive construction project going on in Albuquerque, called "The Big I". This was a rebuilding of the interchanges of Interstate routes 25 and 40. The first nine months of commuting through this every day was long and difficult, but the project was miraculously completed ahead of schedule. After completion, commuting from Bernalillo to the VA was easy.

My arrival at the VA was known for about a year. During that time, I naively thought the VA would have prepared a proper office for me. I was given a key to a small room currently being occupied by two of my residents. We had only one computer among the three of us, and each of us had a small desk. There was a door to a bathroom that we were locked out of.

IS's office was on the other side, and he claimed it as his private bathroom. Having just come from a beautiful private office in Ithaca, I was quite annoyed at not having my own private office. It was unusual for an attending doctor to share office space with his residents, but I soon learned that space at VA Medical Centers was at a premium. I was subsequently moved into two other private offices during my employ as dictated by hospital space needs.

My two office mates were second-year residents (a podiatric residency is three years). They were also practicing Mormons. I learned a great deal about their religion, and grew to respect their faith and beliefs. We got along famously. My home town of Rochester, NY was near where the annual Mormon Pageant was held, which I attended once.

I learned what a "Jack Mormon" is, although neither of them was one.

The first-year residents shared an even more crowded office with fourth-year podiatry students on another floor. All these students and residents were at the top of their classes from the California College of Podiatric Medicine (CCPM) in San Francisco (currently the Samuel Merritt College of Podiatric Medicine), IS's Alma Mater, and hand-picked by him. Only two of these four students would be picked to stay at the VA for the first two years of their three-year residency.

According to IS, CCPM was the only podiatry school that would allow fourth-year students to spend that year entirely off the CCPM campus in Albuquerque. As an adjunct faculty member of CCPM, IS traveled to the College twice a year to interview students. Since I was also training students and residents, I was appointed as an Adjunct Assistant Professor at the College. I was also interested in visiting the College to be involved in the student selection process, but after initially inviting me, IS never allowed me the opportunity to do so.

I never set foot on that campus. I did have some input regarding the choice of the next years 'residents, since I also supervised them, but IS had the final say. Of the two second year residents, one would stay in Albuquerque at Lovelace Healthcare and the other would go to Kaiser Permanente in Sacramento for their third year. Each program had its particular strengths, and each resident usually got their choice without acrimony.

Podiatry services in the VA are organized under the Surgical Service, headed by the Chief of the Service who is typically an MD surgeon. At the Albuquerque VA, the Podiatry Section was headed by IS with me as an attending podiatrist.

Sections are unofficial designations in the VA, and the section chief's name does not formally appear on any evaluation form. David Peterson, MD was Chief of the Surgical Service. Dave was a general surgeon who was responsible for my formal hiring. Even though IS actually offered me the position, as Chief of the Surgical Service, Dr. Peterson officially wrote me the letter of hire. He was also responsible for supporting my Chief Grade pay rate decided in Cleveland by the Podiatry Standards Board. Dave's wife became friends with Linda, and they went shopping together on several occasions. Dave was a fine fellow, and we got along very well.

Prior to my arrival in Albuquerque, IS had never been invited to any social functions with the Petersons. Dave invited both me and IS and our spouses to their annual Christmas party. Linda and I drove IS and his wife to the party. IS's wife was a Senior Vice-President at the Bank of Albuquerque. She had smoothed the way for our mortgage on the Bernalillo house, and facilitated our ability to close via phone and fax prior to our arrival in New Mexico. She put us in contact with another VP who handled our personal finances. We very much enjoyed dealing with him, and he took good care of our banking needs.

Politics is part and parcel of any work place, but those at the Albuquerque VA were toxic. There was another general surgeon named Steve Frank, who had been passed over for Service Chief in lieu of Dave Peterson. He held a grudge over his non-selection that would soon erupt into considerable unpleasantness for me and others.

Dr. Frank was a body builder with a similar mentality. He was a professional bully who came and left work dressed in tank top and biker shorts, and wore his hair with a buzz cut and ponytail. He would change into scrubs at work. I knew nothing of his surgical abilities.

Within about six to nine months of my arrival, there was reorganization within the VA, and a new title was created, "Manager, Surgical Care Line." The stated purpose of this new position was to integrate all services related to the performance of surgery at a VA hospital to streamline the delivery of surgical care to the veteran patients. This individual had authority over all the Service Chiefs related to the performance of surgery, including Surgical, Nursing, and Anesthesia Services.

Somehow Dr. Frank had manipulated himself into this powerful position. The bad blood between himself and Dave Peterson became evident at a subsequent Surgical Service meeting where Dave said one thing and Steve overrode his authority in front of the entire Service. Dave's father, also a general surgeon, was the past Assistant Dean for Clinical Affairs at the University of New Mexico Health Sciences Center (medical school). Dave applied and was hired for that position, and he soon resigned from the VA to work at the University full time. Dr. Frank soon commandeered Dave's former corner office with sweeping views of Sandia Peak. I did not know it at the time, but IS and Steve had developed a strong relationship. In retrospect, it was crystal clear to me how two bullies could become such good buddies.

I had no direct relationship with Steve Frank. We occasionally walked out of the building together after work and exchanged small talk-he in his biker outfit and me in "normal" clothes. After Dave Peterson left, there were some catastrophic changes within the Surgical Service. Two other general surgeons, including my friend Paul Gleason and another surgeon were both forced to leave the VA by Steve. The entire anesthesiology staff except for the CRNAs (Certified Registered Nurse Anesthetist), including one of my new friends, left and went to the University because of Steve's bullying.

A few months after David Peterson left, J. David Pearl, MD was selected as Acting Chief of the Surgical Service. Dr. Pearl, whom I shall refer to in this narrative as JD, was an orthopedic oncologist. This is a sub-specialty of orthopedics concerned with treating bone cancers. JD was a mild-mannered man, whom I soon discovered was also spineless; quite a poetic description for an orthopedist!

One November day, JD came looking for me in clinic. He motioned me to an empty patient room and proceeded to go over my annual evaluation with me. My annual evaluation was delayed due to the hiatus between the two service chiefs. My initial three-month evaluation by IS was fine.

Linda and I had recently returned from two weeks in Hawaii-the first week being a meeting in Maui of the Northwest Podiatric Foundation located in Seattle. My longtime friend, Marc Kaplan, DPM had invited me to give a lecture at this meeting. Marc was on the Board of Directors of the Foundation and had been living and practicing in the Seattle area since leaving the Army. We became friends in the Army and were colleagues; he at Walter Reed, and me at Fort Meade. Marc showed me how to do my first joint implant. Loyalty has always been one of my strongest attributes, and Marc and I maintained our friendship over the past thirty years, through both our divorces and beyond.

Apparently during my two-week leave from the VA, IS and JD had conspired to fabricate a completely false evaluation of my performance with the ultimate goal of forcing me out of my job. As JD went over the various parts of my evaluation, I was nearly speechless. The VA Proficiency Report is divided up into categories, numbered I-V, concluding in an overall rating. The final item on the form, number nineteen, is a place for comments.

Each category is scored as Unsatisfactory, Low Satisfactory, Satisfactory, High Satisfactory, and Outstanding. In order to "pass", one could not fall below Satisfactory in the overall rating.

First, JD began our session with some introductory comments. He said, "Evan, I realize you are used to getting A's in your courses, and were considered a big shot back in New York. You are probably not used to failure." He continued, "But here, your clinical work is low satisfactory."

I replied, "How can you explain my obvious success up until now?"

He refused to answer me directly, but proceeded directly to the comments part of the report. This section was filled with inaccurate and unproven statements.

JD began with I, Clinical Competence. He said, "You scored Low Satisfactory."

I replied, "How could that be? I've been practicing podiatry for over 25 years."

"I've successfully treated thousands of patients over these years, including many here." He ignored my response and immediately proceeded to Category II, Educational Competence.

"You scored Low Satisfactory on this one." I replied somewhat indignantly, "In addition to my podiatry degree, I have a Masters' degree, and I have published several professional papers in peer-reviewed journals."

He replied, "No comment."

Category III is Research and Development. "You scored Low Satisfactory."

I was stunned. "How could this be?"

He replied, "You haven't done any research here."

I replied, "I didn't know that research was considered part of my job here."

Category IV is Administrative Competence. He said,

"You got a Satisfactory on this one."

Category V is Personal Qualities.

"You scored Low Satisfactory."

I replied, "How can this be, I get along with all the residents, students, nurses, and even the custodial staff. I even considered you and IS my friends."

He said, "No comment."

The key part of the report was the Overall Rating.

"You scored Low Satisfactory."

I asked him if this was his own personal evaluation of my work, and he said, "No, this comes directly from IS."

My immediate reaction was, "If this is not your actual evaluation of my work here, you need to rip this up and start over. It's your signature, not IS's on this form."

His response was predictable, "I'll have to rely on IS, since he is your direct supervisor."

I replied, "He's hardly ever in clinic before 10:30 every morning; I don't think he can adequately judge my clinical skills."

I refused to sign this false evaluation. I knew this was the kiss of death to my career at the Albuquerque VA.

Steve Frank attempted to intimidate me into signing the document, but he was unsuccessful at doing so. I had visited the HR Department on several occasions regarding this matter, and although they were not very helpful, they did tell me I did not have to sign the form if I disagreed with its contents.

Meanwhile, I was still performing all my clinical duties including surgery and was still involved with training the residents. One of IS's unfounded criticisms was in regards to certain surgical techniques. JD agreed to have me work in his office on Friday afternoons using sawbones models in remediation sessions to "refine" my techniques, but Steve Frank vetoed that plan. JD then began to investigate the outcomes of my surgical cases. I said, "You have to compare my outcomes to IS's, otherwise this will be unfair." He reluctantly agreed.

I presented him with published studies stating that there was no reliable way to measure outcomes in foot and ankle surgery, to which he replied that he knew that because he was an orthopedist! Where this was all headed was to the local Professional Standards Board.

A newly hired Title 38 employee is on probation for two years, and does not have the protection that a permanent government employee has after the two years is up. I consulted with my friend, Paul Gleason, MD who was also having his own issues with Dr. Frank. Paul told me that as long as they still let me see, treat, and operate on patients, they must not really be concerned about my clinical competence. While I appreciated Paul's support, it gave me small comfort. It soon became clear my professional reputation was at stake.

There is nothing more valuable to a professional than their reputation. For the previous twenty-five years, I had enjoyed a good reputation among my peers, my patients, and my professional societies. As described in the previous chapter, I had just been appointed to the Board of Podiatry for the State of New York-one of the highlights of my career. Now this was all at risk due to IS's petty jealousy.

IS perceived himself as superior to me as a podiatrist, and was insanely jealous that I had been invited to be a guest speaker at the Maui meeting instead of him. He refused to let me go to another meeting regarding a new antibiotic, and berated me as "some hick from Upstate New York." Yet, he hired me fully knowing all my strengths and limitations. I later learned he hired me over two other very well respected and internationally known podiatrists who also had applied for my job. IS knew his ego (and possibly his continued position as Chief) could not stand the competition with either of those outstanding doctors.

My predecessor only lasted about six months as an attending. She was one of IS's residents who was bullied, intimidated and sexually harassed by him. I had not met her until I began speaking with her by phone near the end of my tenure at the VA. Had I known what she had been through, I would have done things differently.

With my professional reputation at risk, I suspected I needed legal advice. I called my cousin Steve (a senior partner in a large

Washington law firm) who quickly confirmed my need for legal representation. I finally located Gary Richards who was a partner in a large Albuquerque law firm. He specialized in representing professionals in such matters. The very first thing he said to me was, "If you are here to have me fight for your job, I can't help you. I can only help you protect your professional reputation."

After several sessions with Gary, he agreed to accompany me to my meeting with the Chief-of-Staff. The Chief-of-Staff did not allow Gary into the meeting, but I reviewed the content with him after that meeting. The Chief-of-Staff was a psychiatrist, and my previous interactions with him had been just superficial elevator talk.

I was able to persuade JD to allow me to stay until I found another position. He convinced Steve Frank to agree to this, although IS wanted me gone immediately.

JD really felt badly about how things snowballed, and tried to find me another VA position somewhere else. However, I fault him as Acting Chief of Surgical Service, for not having the courage to stand up to IS, who was his subordinate. Dave Peterson would not have allowed IS to get away with his antics. I guess the corporate culture was one that did not want to have such acrimony in the Surgical Service; therefore, I had to go. I knew I had the support of others at the VA, including the Chief of Orthopedics, the Surgical Service quality management nurse, and others.

The Orthopedic Chief complemented me on training such fine residents, who told me, "Your podiatry residents stand shoulder to shoulder with my orthopedic residents."

I had applied for the Chief-of-Podiatry position at the Fayetteville, Arkansas VAMC, and was pursued by them. I worried that if I accepted that job and started there, I could still be terminated if my bogus evaluation somehow surfaced and my two years were not completed at that point.

I avoided IS as much as possible during my final months at the VA. Our only interactions were unpleasant and acrimonious. He gave me a hard time about taking sick leave for doctor's appointments and for going to the HR department. He wanted me gone and out of his sight. He became very angry and threatening on several occasions, and if I knew then what I now know about harassment in the workplace, I might have been able to successfully fight for my job using that approach. I was still six months away from completing the two-year probation period, and IS was keenly aware of that timetable. I did explore EEO options, but had no grounds to file a complaint under that venue. Other than Gary Richards, I had no "big brother" in my corner to advise me on strategy. In retrospect, I do not believe Gary was aggressive enough in handling my case. I now believe he or someone else more experienced in these matters could have assisted me in fighting for my job.

* * *

Most people can remember where they were on the morning of September 11, 2001. I was just leaving my house in Bernalillo for work, listening to NPR radio in the car, when I heard of the first plane strike into the World Trade Center. The announcers were uncertain at that point if this was an accidental event. By the time I got to the VA, the second plane had struck the second tower, and terrorism was now a fact. Within days of that tragedy, all VA employees had to show their badge from their cars to the VA Police before being allowed to park.

* * *

I can recall my relief and jubilation at beginning this job at the VA-relief from the tribulations of private practice, and the joy of returning to education after so many years from my first teaching job at a two-year branch of the State University of New York at Canton. I can also remember smiling from ear-to-ear as I drove to work in the bright sunshine, almost incredulous that I was actually being paid to enjoy myself. IS initially presented himself as a laid-back Californian, who initially allowed me to find my own rhythm and pace in my new job. We had much in common. He was a former ski instructor and his first wife was Jewish. He came from a wealthy family in the Los Angeles area. He idolized his deceased father who had owned a prosperous auto dealership. I met his mother once while she was visiting IS-a small, quiet woman. The IS's had no children, and the residents were the closest he had to his own kids. He was generous with gifts, but stingy on praise, and he had his favorites. One of them had just finished his residency before I arrived, and went back to his home state of Florida to practice.

His father had been an orthopedic surgeon, and he went back to his hometown to practice. He was dating a woman from Albuquerque who was a social worker at the VA. They eventually got married, and moved back to Albuquerque. He was immediately hired at Presbyterian Hospital as an employed podiatrist-a job I had also applied for. His co-resident was also working at Presbyterian as well as his wife, an internist. I had no such connections. The newly hired podiatrist at Presbyterian was IS's surrogate son, and both enjoyed fly fishing. IS took an annual trip to northern New Mexico to one of Ted Turner's exclusive private hunting and fishing camps with private lakes. He took his newly minted resident as his guest.

My weekly work week consisted in supervising the residents in clinic in the mornings, and making rounds on inpatients in the afternoons, with one morning a week for my surgical cases. I was allowed one half-day a week as administrative time to take care of the various tasks necessary to sustain a government career. On Friday mornings, I supervised the PACT (Prevention of Amputation Care and Treatment) Clinic while IS was in surgery. To my consternation, he usually scheduled his most advanced cases for that day, so I was only able to observe the afternoon cases after PACT Clinic. Before hiring me, IS had offered to train me on surgeries I was unable to learn in New York due to that state's limited scope of practice at the time. An early warning sign I failed to notice was his lack of commitment to that initial promise.

IS's chronic tardiness was either overlooked or ignored by his supervisors- for what reason I never understood. On one Friday morning, his surgical patient was in the OR with the residents ready to go, but IS had not yet arrived. I was called from PACT Clinic to attend the case, but it was a surgery I was not familiar with. That day's operating room schedule was delayed until IS wandered in.

I arose early on the morning of March 31, and put on a tie and jacket for the second and last time for work. It was a cool, crisp day in early spring, with the classic azure blue New Mexico sky and no humidity. I had never lived in such a great climate as I found in New Mexico. I'd never felt so well physically since living in that climate. Most of my aches and pains were diminished. Mornings always reminded me of crisp fall days back East.

After arriving at the VA, I proceeded with the task of clearing station; checking out of Human Resources, signing papers, and receiving a copy of my personnel records. Suspiciously, and probably fortunately there was no evidence of the unsigned bogus evaluation in my official records.

The months preceding my departure from the Albuquerque VA was spent in an intensive job search. I was about to start a new private practice in my hometown of Bernalillo, but I knew it would be years before that practice could sustain us. Aside from the possible opportunity at the Fayetteville VA, my only other firm job offer was from a private practice in Santa Fe which I accepted with reluctance but out of necessity.

Drs. Mike Allen and Stan Gorman were partners in Northern New Mexico Foot Care based in Santa Fe. They had satellite offices in Espanola and Taos, as well as contracts with local Indian Health centers in Santa Fe and Cochiti Pueblo. Mike and Stan had been equal partners since 1976, and had recently lost a female associate who became an Army podiatrist (she recently retired from the Army as a Lieutenant Colonel). My new job entailed much driving around northern New Mexico to service these satellite offices. Once every two months, I made the trip to an outlying clinic in Tierra Amarilla near the Colorado border, a round trip of three hundred twenty miles from home in one day.

My starting pay was only seventy-five thousand dollars, but there were bonus incentives for productivity as well as a promise for future partnership written into my contract. I was tired of private practice, but this was my only firm job offer. Gorman was two years older, and Allen was one year younger than me. Gorman was looking to retire in about a year, opening up the possibility of my buying out his interest in the partnership. My start day was May first.

I had a month from the time I left the VA until starting my new job. I was mentally exhausted and depressed over the recent turn of events in my life, and welcomed the month's respite between jobs. Fortunately, Linda convinced me to pay off the mortgage on our Bernalillo home with the remainder of the proceeds from the Ithaca practice sale.

The next day, we loaded up the dogs and drove to Telluride, Colorado for a week of skiing. Due to various health problems, Linda could no longer ski. She busied herself with relaxing with the dogs and reading as we stayed at a pet-friendly slope side condo. We explored the town after I returned from the slopes, and dined at local restaurants.

Telluride is a picturesque old mining town situated at the end of a box canyon deep within Colorado's San Juan Mountains. It was difficult to get to, but worth the trip. The skiing and scenery were fantastic. The drive from Durango to Silverton and Ouray on the way to Telluride was spectacular, and definitely not for flatlander drivers.

Linda had never been to San Antonio, Texas, so we decided to take another road trip to that destination. Skiing had given me a temporary euphoria, and the long car trip to San Antonio gave us much time to talk and reflect about recent events. I was clearly depressed about what had happened at the VA and was not looking forward to returning to private practice as an employee.

May first soon approached, and my work schedule was: Monday and Wednesday at the Espanola office. Tuesday morning at the Santa Fe Indian Hospital where my new employers had a contract to provide podiatric services for one morning per week. Tuesday afternoon in surgery at the Santa Fe Regional Medical Center; Thursday in Taos. I was off most Fridays unless I had another surgery or one of the other doctors requested my assistance in surgery.

This sounds like a reasonable schedule until you factor in the driving distances. Bernalillo is about eighty miles one way from Espanola with Santa Fe on the way there at about forty-five miles. Taos is another forty-five miles past Espanola. My new employer paid for my lodging in Taos every Wednesday evening along with meal allotments and gas money. After I finished work at about 5 pm on Thursday in Taos, I had a two-hour drive home into the blinding setting sun.

One day after arriving at the remote outpost of Tierra Amarilla, my assistant realized she had forgotten our instruments we needed for the day. We called the Santa Fe office, and were met half way by another assistant who handed off the instruments. While on the way, driving at eighty mph, I struck a coyote that ran across the road. Me, and my assistant, were fine, but the coyote and my SUV were not. I had a large dent in my plastic bumper. I later asked Mike, the managing partner if he would reimburse my deductible for the damage, since it happened during a company trip, and he refused to do so.

The one saving grace about all this driving was that it happened in scenic northern New Mexico. The drive from Espanola to Taos is through the striking Taos canyon along a beautiful mountain river. The drive from Espanola to Tierra Amarilla runs through the Brazos rock formations-both colorful and geologically interesting. In Tierra Amarilla, on a clear day one can appreciate distant views of several of southern Colorado's 14,000-foot peaks near Alamosa. Traffic was sparse and aside from a few bad winter days, the weather was nearly always sunny and dry.

Most of the time I relished the solitude of driving, listening to CDs of the Mamas and the Papas, Handel's Coronation Anthems, and barbershop quartet tunes. I sang with the Ithaca Barbershop Chorus prior to leaving for New Mexico. I found this music soothing and uplifting in an otherwise depressing situation.

I also had many self-dialogues, and concluded I needed to find a different work situation as soon as possible. Espanola is situated in a valley west of the snow-capped Sangre de Christo Mountains. That office was a block away from a public park. I would quickly eat my lunch in the office and then spend the rest of my lunch hour walking at the park and admiring the mountain scenery and sunshine. Allen and Gorman owned the building, and had recently moved in from an office at the local hospital across the street. The building was just renovated, but the heating system was faulty. The employees and I had to wear our coats all winter indoors while treating patients. It was definitely not a good place to work.

Espanola was ninety-five percent Hispanic, and was considered to be the heroin capital of the country. Drug seeking patients were common, and I was the new doc in town. I had several patients visit me with vague complaints of pain. It was clear that they were really drug seekers. I was not going to be the new "Candy Man" in town.

I did have one patient who had sustained a serious foot injury, and her need for pain medication was legitimate. Podiatrists do not treat chronic pain, and I referred such patients in need of chronic medications to their primary doctor or to a special pain clinic for long term management. I called this patient's family doctor and asked him if he would manage this particular patient's pain medication. He said, "I'd rather not, but I can see why you would not be the one to do it. I'll have her sign a pain contract and I'll manage her chronic pain."

He called me a week later to tell me, "The patient's husband was arrested by the DEA for selling her pain meds on the street."

I was exhausted from the week's work, driving, and the stress of being in a situation I did not really want to be in. On Friday and Saturday, I began my own private practice in the office of a local nurse practitioner just around the corner from my house. Bernalillo is an old Hispanic town and a northern suburb of Albuquerque. The area was rapidly growing, and the nearest podiatrist was over ten miles away.

The nurse practitioner had a small, poorly laid out office, but promised to refer me all her patients in need of podiatric care. I completed all the paperwork necessary to participate with the local insurance companies, and obtained surgical privileges at two local hospitals in Albuquerque. Of course, I still remained on staff at the hospitals in Santa Fe and Espanola. I was able to purchase some basic equipment used such as an x-ray machine and processor from a local retiring podiatrist.

Having been in my own private practice in Ithaca for nineteen years, I knew the tremendous marketing effort and time involved in starting a new practice. The nurse practitioner, my landlord charged me a nominal rent for one cramped exam room, and let me use her office staff. Unfortunately, her staff was completely inept, and not motivated to assist me. This may have something to do with the fact that I could not afford to pay them yet! I lost most of the few dollars I earned by unfiled insurance claims.

As it turned out, my landlord only had a handful of patients who needed my services, so I did the usual things to promote myself: Speaking to groups, newspaper ads, and distributing flyers. I also personally met all the primary care doctors in my area, and handed them my new business cards.

While I worked Monday-Thursday for Northern New Mexico Foot Care, the staff in Bernalillo would make the few appointments for me on Friday and Saturday.

One of the highlights of my time in New Mexico was connecting with an old friend from Ithaca. Dr. Jerry H. was a family doctor who sold his Ithaca practice in the mid-1990s and went to work for the U.S. State Department. He became the doctor for the diplomats and their families in places like Buenos Ares. He and his wife, Joanne loved to travel.

We kept in loose contact after leaving Ithaca, and Jerry knew I was somewhere in New Mexico.

During the early days of my employment my new employers paid for lodging Tuesday night in Santa Fe to minimize my commute the next day to Espanola. One evening after work, the phone rang in my motel room. "Hello, is this Meltzer?"

It was a strange but familiar voice. "Is this really H?"

Jerry and I had a weekly date to play racquetball when we both lived in Ithaca. It was a ritual, and we were closely matched. After our game, he would always ask, "Meltzer, are you ready for a steam?"

We would always head to the steam room after our match, but our ritual always included his asking the same question every week. Jerry and I became close friends, and I considered him a mentor in practice and business matters.

I had adopted an authoritative attitude from treating soldiers at Fort Meade, and soon found that this approach was not popular among civilians. I met Jerry through a cousin and I learned through Jerry the concept of the doctor-patient partnership that I continued until my retirement.

Jerry left his position at the State Department because they were going to send him to Islamabad. He would not be allowed to have Joanne join him, so he left that agency. He was hired as the Medical Director of the Santa Clara Pueblo Indian Health Center, just outside of Espanola, New Mexico only two miles from my Espanola office-what a wonderful coincidence! He was renting a small casita in downtown Santa Fe while Joanne was finishing up her job in Washington, D.C.

We met for lunch at a Mexican restaurant between our offices and renewed our friendship. He graciously allowed me to sleep on my air mattress on the floor of his tiny casita on Tuesday nights. One day, we actually car pooled to work. What are the chances of two old friends from Ithaca, New York car-pooling from Santa Fe to Espanola, New Mexico? I was able to stay with Jerry on Tuesday evenings until Joanne moved from Washington.

We had a wonderful time together.

One day while working in the Espanola office, I felt like meeting Jerry for lunch. I called his office and was told, "Dr. H doesn't work here anymore."

Jerry had always been a private person, and when I finally caught up with him, he never really told me what had happened. I knew he and the Clinic Director did not get along well, but was unaware of the seriousness of their disagreements.

Jerry and Joanne were also looking for real estate in Santa Fe; in fact, we were sort of competing with each other in that endeavor. Fortunately for them, while they came close to buying a house, they did not. Jerry managed to a get temporary *locum tenens* job for a few weeks out of state.

The last time I saw him was when he stayed overnight at our home in Bernalillo on his way driving to Dallas. He had just accepted a permanent full-time job as a civilian Army doctor in Vicenza, Italy. I never found out the true reasons behind Jerry's dismissal from Santa Clara.

The long-distance driving was wearing on me, and I would come home exhausted. My employers were encouraging me to move to either Santa Fe or Taos. Linda and I put our house on the market, and started looking at real estate in Taos. Like most of the towns in Northern New Mexico, Taos was old and predominantly Hispanic. It has charm, and a world class ski area. Donald Rumsfeld, Ted Turner and Julia Roberts lived there. While we loved the scenery and the surrounding area, we felt it was too remote considering Linda's health problems. We began our foray into the Santa Fe real estate market.

The capital city of New Mexico, population about sixty thousand at that time, is situated at an elevation of seven thousand feet above sea level, at the base of the Sangre de Christo Mountains. Santa Fe prides itself as the "City Different." It was rumored to have the second largest number of artist studios outside of New York City. Santa Fe is a charming place to visit, but a very expensive city in which to live. The City Council voted to raise the minimum wages to ten dollars an hour for all businesses having over twenty-five employees to help with their living expenses in Santa Fe.

We soon learned that our half-million dollar plus home in Bernalillo with twenty-four hundred square feet would be priced about a third higher if it were located in Santa Fe. It was not difficult to find some beautiful homes in Santa Fe, but they were clearly out of our price range.

One weekend we attended the Santa Fe Parade of Homes, and toured the million dollar plus homes just for fun. We saw one hilltop home priced at thirteen million, complete with a wine cellar, wine tasting room, media room, etc.

There was a brand-new Cadillac Escalade in the garage with a red ribbon around it included as a gift from the seller to the new buyer. This was a third home for a Houston oil family with a prominent photo of their family on top of the piano standing with the George H. W. Bush family. We were told that Gene Hackman's land was visible from the balcony of that house. On another trip to Santa Fe, we were nearly run over by Ali McGraw as she was backing her large SUV out of a parking space. As long as I am dropping names, Val Kilmer owned a ranch near Pecos, east of Santa Fe. Robert Redford is also a property owner in the area.

No doubt, these celebrities help contribute to the high cost of living in Santa Fe. Jane Fonda and Don Imus also lived in the area.

Fortunately, we had a purchase contract on our Bernalillo fall through. We would have lost about a hundred thousand dollars if it had gone through. Linda and I finally decided to move into a rental house in Santa Fe, and rent out the Bernalillo home.

Our life outside of my work was adventurous and fulfilling. We lived in an upscale gated community in Bernalillo situated along the Rio Grande River called Bosque Encantado De C 'de Baca. Neither of us spoke Spanish, and we joked that the name of our community meant "Mosquito infested swamp." It actually means, "Enchanted Forest." The C 'de Baca family had owned the land for generations. Our home was among the smallest of the Phase I homes, situated on a full acre of land. The million-dollar plus homes were larger and most were located right on the river bank.

Ours was a Silver Award winner in its price range in the Albuquerque Parade of Homes, and featured large windows with sweeping views of Sandia Peak to the east. Since all the homes here were built on the river's flood plain, all had to be built upon raised pads of earth brought in to each home site. Soon after we moved in, one of our neighbors who was a builder told us our pad was inadequate.

We paid to have another sixty-five cubic yards of earth trucked from a sand hill across the street from the development, and graded around our property. That property is now a fully developed gated community.

Water is a scarce and valuable commodity in the desert southwest. Most homes are landscaped with xeriscape features, meaning mostly stone and not grass. I received a permit from the state engineer's office for five dollars to have an irrigation well drilled on our property. We were on city water and sewer services otherwise. We landscaped our home with gravel, large moss rocks collected by us from the Santa Fe National Forest, and appropriate desert plants and trees. We also planted a small vegetable garden and grape vines.

All of this was watered from our well as drip irrigation. We spent well over a hundred-thousand-dollars for this elaborate landscape even with our doing much of the work ourselves. The grounds were beautiful as a result of Linda's artistic landscaping ability and no doubt contributed to the eventual sale of the house.

During one of the contractor phases of our landscaping project, the foreman was away from the job. The project was dragging along, and we were anxious to have it finished. The foreman had told us earlier it would be finished "mañana". One day as Linda saw the workers slacking off, she decided to take action. She carried the cordless phone outside, and proceeded to have the following conversation into the phone. She made sure the workers were within earshot.

"My husband just bought me a Lady Smith and Wesson .38 caliber pistol. Can you please tell me a good place to go for target practice?"

"Ok, thank you."

The phone was never turned on, but the workers who overheard this imaginary conversation scampered to their tools and shovels faster than we'd ever seen them move before.

The project was finished on time and within budget.

We enjoyed an active social life in the community. Most neighbors were our age, some retired, some still working. We were probably among the least well off financially, but were universally liked and respected. One house down the street was owned by a prosperous male couple. They threw lavish parties, complete with valet parking (we walked), top shelf liquor, tents in the back yard and live entertainment.

We socialized with our other friends and neighbors on a regular basis, at our house, theirs, and informally while walking around the development.

Our house was at the perimeter of the development, adjacent to the Sandoval County Sherriff's Posse rodeo grounds.

Many years ago, this facility was in what was then rural Sandoval County. Now it is surrounded by housing developments. We spent many wakeful weekend nights listening to loud music, traffic, drunks and cowboys. The bright stadium lights would shine into our bedroom window until the wee hours.

Prior to leaving for Texas, the Leland Cypress trees we planted grew tall enough to block out most of this distraction. The Sherriff's Posse was offered millions of dollars for their property from developers as incentive to move out further, but they declined. Their typical Hispanic response was, "We were here first, and you gringos will just have to put up with it."

There was a book published that described the one thousand things you must do before you die, similar to the "Bucket List". One of those is to see the Albuquerque International Balloon Fiesta.

Albuquerque is situated in the Rio Grande River valley just west of Sandia Peak. This geographical condition causes winds to circulate in a box-like pattern, with the air mass blocked by Sandia Peak to the east. This makes for an ideal air movement pattern for hot air balloons. The Balloon Fiesta is always the first full week in October, and we went every year we were there.

During our first balloon fiesta, soon after moving into our new home, Linda said one Sunday morning, "Evan, there's a hot air balloon over our back yard!"

We went outside, and the balloonists asked permission to land in the lot next to us. They were hovering only about thirty feet above us. Linda jokingly said, "What would you like for breakfast?"

Bernalillo is at the northern edge of the box-like air mass pattern, and many balloons were landing all in and around our development-an incredible sight. One morning while Linda was in the shower she heard a "woosh" and saw a balloon full of people outside the bathroom window. Later, Linda said, "We'd better keep our bedroom blinds closed during the balloon fiesta."

The Balloon Fiesta Park is located due south of Bernalillo in Albuquerque. In the early mornings, one can watch the mass ascension-the launching of hundreds of colorful hot air balloons of all whimsical shapes and sizes. At night, the spectators can marvel at the balloon afterglow, where all the tethered balloons fire their burners at once after a countdown. The bright shapes and colors light up in spectacular fashion.

Until 2002, the Fiesta was sponsored by my hometown company and former summer job employer, Eastman Kodak. More film was shot during that event than at any other single event in the world. Kodak ended their sponsorship as digital photography became popular. As is now well known and mentioned in my introduction, Kodak is significantly downsized. They invented digital photography but failed to capitalize on their invention.

The weather is not always cooperative during early October. Participants and spectators travel great distances to attend, and sometimes the wind and rain do not cooperate. During one Fiesta, a balloon strayed into Kirtland Air Force Base's restricted air space. The balloon pilots were apprehended by the Air Force police.

During our last Fiesta until my retirement, a balloon carrying a fifty-six-year-old pilot and two young boys crashed into a cell tower during high winds. Later that same day, Linda and I parked at a place just south of the Balloon Fiesta Park to watch the balloons. Linda said, "Evan, what's that attached to that tall tower over there twisting in the wind?"

I looked over to where she was pointing, and said, "It looks like a deflated balloon."

At that point, we had not heard about the accident.

Linda said, "I hope no one was hurt or killed."

I replied, "That's a very long distance to fall from."

Later that evening, the local TV news networks were interviewing the balloon pilot and his young passengers. The pilot was a hero as he was able to talk the boys down the tower as they climbed down together. Both the pilot and boys were unhurt.

* * *

The state of New Mexico is blessed with abundant mineral resources. There is active copper and silver mining in the southwestern portion of the state, and New Mexico Tech in Socorro graduates mining engineers and has a fine mineral collection and museum.

We joined the Albuquerque Gem and Mineral Club that met once a month at the Natural History Museum in old town Albuquerque. The Club sponsors a field trip each month at various locations around the state and sometimes in neighboring states. Each meeting had renowned collectors show slides and specimens from their collecting trips.

When I was a boy growing up in Rochester, New York, I attended similar meetings at the Rochester Academy of Sciences, Mineral Section, also held at the local museum. I became interested in rocks and minerals at an early age. My childhood mineral collection moved with me from my parent's house to my various residences in Ithaca. One day, Linda asked me, "Would you consider selling or donating your collection so we don't have to keep moving it around?"

I was able to sell the collection on eBay.

I broke my leg playing sandlot football when I was thirteen years old. I happened to mention my interest in rocks and minerals to the nurse at the orthopedist's office. She said she had a son who was also quite interested in minerals. Mrs. Pinch invited me to meet her son, Bill at their home. Bill Pinch lived with his mother in a modest apartment not too far from my house.

The apartment complex had storage rooms, and the Pinch's was filled with custom wooden cabinets filled with beautiful mineral specimens, all organized according to Dana's System of Minerology and neatly labeled with Bill's personal labels. Bill was several years older than me, and during his first year of college at the University of New Mexico in Albuquerque, he was badly injured in a fall while collecting minerals. He had to drop out of college because of his injuries.

The place where this accident happened was called Blanchard Claims, near the two- building town of Bingham, New Mexico, not far from the Trinity Site where the first atomic bomb was detonated in July, 1945. Mrs. Blanchard, a widow, held the claims to the lead mines on her property. Apparently, Bill was able to charm his way into letting him collect there. Since that time, Blanchard Claims has become a world class mineral location and a classic Dana location for some one-of-a kind minerals. As a kid, I was awed by the beauty and rarity of Bill's specimens from Blanchard, and vowed that I would collect there myself one day.

Mrs. Blanchard has long since died, but there is a rock shop in Bingham that sells some examples of the local minerals, including radioactive glass called "Trinitite" from the original atomic explosion at the Trinity Site. The claims are now owned and worked for mineral collecting by several current members of the Albuquerque Gem and Mineral Club. We had the privilege of going there for one of our field trips, and collected some pristine crystals from the Sunshine Number Three mine. We also collected at a gold mine (no gold found), hunted for turquoise, and collected garnets all on separate trips to other parts of the state.

I should also say that Linda loved doing this as much if not more than me. We decorated our xeriscape in Bernalillo with "yard rocks"; those large pieces not quite specimen quality but colorful none the less.

For my birthday, Linda wanted to "buy" me a gold mine. We traveled to the Bureau of Land Management office in Santa Fe, where they provide maps with sites available for staking claims. The rules have not changed since the Mining Act of 1872. This law allowed private citizens to stake a claim and mine on public lands. One of the Act's stipulations state that the claimholder must show some sort of mining activity expending at least one-hundred-dollars per year (that fee has subsequently increased) to maintain the claim. One could not erect a permanent dwelling on the claim, just mining structures. Modern day interceded with our plans, as we also learned that the claim holder could be held liable if someone was injured on the claim site. BLM land is still public and trespassing is legal. Although it would have been a unique gift, we abandoned the idea. Most of the best-known mineral collecting localities were already claimed by others.

Since leaving New Mexico, we've moved our boxes of specimens to Texas, Montana and Mississippi without opening them. It seems that we have not felt permanent in one place or had the proper shelving to display them to open the boxes.

Bill Pinch became a world-famous mineralogist. At one time, he probably had one of the finest private mineral collections in the world. He stayed in the Rochester area, got married and moved into a large home. My children had the distinct privilege of meeting him and viewing his collection. My parents kept in touch with Bill, occasionally buying an opal or other gem from him.

I knew nothing about diamonds, and when I asked for Linda's hand in marriage, I called Bill for diamond advice. He procured a beautiful stone at a good price that I had set in a ring by a life-long jeweler friend of my parents.

A sizeable portion of Bill's private collection consisted of highly radioactive minerals from Africa. Bill's wife was uncomfortable with having them in their home. Bill eventually sold his collection 1989 to the Canadian Museum of Nature for $3.5 million US dollars (source: williampinch.com).

Most mineral names end with the suffix, "ite". One of the greatest honors that can be bestowed upon a mineralogist is to have one named after him. Bill discovered a new specimen by x-ray crystallography, and it was named, "Pinchite" in his honor. Bill is now deceased, but I recently had a nice communication with his son.

* * *

The business aspect of private practice in New Mexico was no different than practicing anywhere. It was all about patient volume, procedures and income. Northern New Mexico Foot Care was a big business, and they had a full-time business manager who focused on the bottom line. I was initially told that I had full authority to make business decisions when I was working alone in the respective offices. Having successfully run my own practice in Ithaca for nineteen years, I had strong opinions and good ideas in these matters. I also learned that two of their loyal employees acted as spies, often undermining my policies.

On Tuesday mornings, I drove from my home to Santa Fe. I stopped at the office there to pick up instruments to take to the Indian Hospital. Mike Allen would often call me into his office to review my production figures and discuss ways at increasing them. I soon dreaded these sessions, because it seemed that no matter how hard I worked, he wanted more productivity. I also had some ethical questions regarding the practice's creative coding policies to increase insurance reimbursement. I would hurry back from the Indian Hospital and go across the street to St. Vincent Hospital (now St. Vincent-Christus Regional Medical Center) with Mike to do three or four surgical cases. We would grab a quick lunch at the hospital cafeteria (their treat) visit with other doctors and then go into surgery for the afternoon.

Mike Allen was a competent surgeon, and either I assisted him or he assisted me, depending upon whose patient it was. Of course, in the beginning of my employ, they were mostly his patients. Assistant surgeons are permitted to bill for their services when there are no resident programs available in the area. I mentioned this to Mike and the business manager and asked them to keep track of this so my billings would be counted towards a possible bonus.

I never worked regularly in their main Santa Fe office. Stan and Mike covered that office exclusively, as they both lived in Santa Fe. I would just stop there on Tuesdays and would also ferry supplies and paperwork to the other offices. Mike was a member of the New Mexico State Board of Podiatry. He personally knew then-Governor Bill Richardson. One day he told me, "I'm embarrassed; I'm short of continuing education credits for my license renewal and I have to go to a meeting as soon as possible."

It didn't look particularly good to have a state board member short of credits.

I saw patients in the Santa Fe office while Mike was away. One of his loyal employee spies reported to Mike a conversation she overheard me having with a patient. It was taken out of context, and upon his return, Mike berated me for it.

The other employee spy lived in Taos, and was the long-time manager of the part-time Taos office. In my opinion, she was the main cause of revenue loss from that office, as many of the patients in that small town were either her family or friends. She would regularly "forget" to collect insurance co-pays or file the proper forms, yet I was often blamed for the lack of production from that office. When I brought this up with Stan and Mike, it was politely ignored.

Early in my employ, Stan announced his retirement early. He had a health problem that was interfering with his ability to practice. This put the subject of partnership on the fast track. Mike asked me to buy out Stan's interest in the practice. Since I had no idea what this was worth, I asked for copies of their books. They did provide this information and I reviewed it with my accountant. During the intervening time that I was considering the purchase, Mike announced, "I bought half of Stan's interest in the practice, leaving you with twenty five percent if you want it."

Owning a minority interest in a business is like owning a fractional ownership of a race horse. You don't get to ride it or direct it where to race. I told Mike, "I'm not interested in sharing just twenty five percent of the profits, with no say in the administration of the practice- thanks but no thanks."

I was working under a one-year employment contract, potentially renewable after the first year. I would have become vested in their pension and profit-sharing plan after one year.

On April fool's Day, I was working in Taos. Mike called me; "Evan, please stop by the Santa Fe office on your way home." I asked him what he wanted, and he just repeated himself. I didn't think much about it, since I would often stop by there anyway to drop off instruments for cleaning and bills for processing. I had a key to that office, and would arrive at night after they had left and drop off the stuff. I remember stopping along the road on the way home that day to buy a bird house for Linda from a roadside vendor.

When I arrived in Santa Fe, it was after 6pm and both Stan and Mike were there. That in itself was an ominous sign.

I said, "Hello."

Mike said, "Evan, give me your office keys."

"Are you serious?"

"Yes."

"Stan, do you agree also?"

"Yes, I'm with Mike. Things have just felt uncomfortable and not right for awhile."

"Can I ask the reasons why you are letting me go?"

Mike said, "It just doesn't feel like the right fit."

After a few more uncomfortable minutes, Mike said, "I'll pay you a month's severance pay since I realize this is sudden and puts you in a tough financial position, but I believe this decision is best for us."

I left the office stunned.

Podiatry was a profession that had often criticized for "Eating its young." Certain members of the profession also "Eat their old" as well.

I had been forced out of a job at the VA, and now fired from a private practice. Ironically, my sister and brother-in law were arriving the next day from Philadelphia for a visit.

The good news was while we lost a deposit on a rental house in Santa Fe and canceled the movers, we still had our beautiful paid-for home in Bernalillo. My only remaining livelihood was my fledgling practice in Bernalillo. I contacted another attorney who assisted me with the original employment contract, and there was some letter writing back and forth. I believe the reason they let me go was because I was not willing to buy into the remaining twenty-five percent of the practice.

I also believe they did not want me to be included in the pension and profit-sharing plan I would have been entitled to after a year of employment (I was one month shy of the year). I also never received any bonus money or portion of the surgical assistant fees I had been promised. I decided it was not worth spending any more in legal fees to fight those issues.

The spring and summer months were filled with a massive project at home. I would work about one-and-a-half days a week in my own practice, because I had so few patients. The rest of the time, Linda and I worked in our one-acre yard hand sifting every square inch of gravel through a sifter I made. We had our drip irrigation replaced, and the contractors left a mess of dirt over the gravel. We were also on the Atkins diet that summer. Between the intense daily exercise and diet, Linda and I dropped a lot of weight. The hard physical labor was good for my body and soul. We joked that this was Linda's "work hardening program." As of this writing, her program is still active and I am the charter member.

Every few days when I was not in the office, my cell phone would ring with a call from my office. "Would you mind coming to the office to see a patient?"

I would quickly shed my dirty clothes, jump into the shower and drive the five minutes to the office. In some ways, it was a nice life, but it wasn't paying the bills.

Once again, Linda's wise decision to pay off the mortgage saved us financially.

I was in the process of looking for a second office in a more populated area of Albuquerque or Rio Rancho when the call came from Staffcare about the job at Fort Hood.

Chapter Three

Fort Hood

"Home of America's Hammer"

2004-2005

It was a disastrous year financially for the Meltzer family. Our taxable income for 2004 was only twenty-four thousand dollars. My good friend from the Albuquerque VA, Paul Gleason, MD had opened my eyes to the world of locum tenens possibilities. Locum tenens is a term used to describe temporary work in the medical field. There are large staffing companies who specialize in placing doctors and nurses in temporary positions. Throughout the spring and summer of 2004, I sent my curriculum vitae to a number of these agencies, including Staffcare. Because podiatry is such a specialized field, there were very few opportunities available. It was crystal clear that my fledgling practice in Bernalillo was failing.

If I had been thirty-five years old and had the patience to wait for patients, I believe I could have eventually succeeded. In fact, I was actively working with a commercial realtor in seeking a second office location in Albuquerque with the idea of also keeping the low-cost Bernalillo location open. I was close to finalizing a lease agreement on office space when I received a phone call from Staffcare, a locum tenens company located in the Dallas area. They asked me, "Are you interested in a locum tenens position to work in the podiatry clinic at Fort Hood, Texas?" I replied,

"What is creating this opportunity?" They answered, "The job is to cover for the active-duty podiatrists who are deployed to Iraq, and is funded by GWOT (Global War On Terrorism)."

"How long does this job last?"

They answered, "The job is for one year, but would be renewable indefinitely because GWOT is not expected to end anytime soon."

I asked, "Could I receive a longer-term contract in writing?"

"Since you only have to give us thirty days notice if you wanted to terminate, Staffcare cannot give you more than one year at a time."

Their explanation seemed reasonable to me. The job paid seventy-five dollars per hour, with more available for call. It also paid for a rental car and housing. There was no health insurance, retirement or any other benefits offered. I was paid a gross salary and was responsible for my own withholding taxes.

Once again, Linda's decision to pay off the mortgage on our Bernalillo home proved to be a wise one. We were in dire financial straits, and might have lost the home if we had to make mortgage payments. I really had little choice but to accept the job and leave my failing practice in New Mexico. Since we believed this job would last indefinitely, and housing was paid for, Linda decided we should buy a home in Texas rather than rent. We also had three dogs at the time, and could not find anyone willing to rent us a home in the Killeen area. One of our good friends in Bernalillo was originally from the Houston area. She told us, "Killeen is the armpit of Texas".

I had heard that before from others who lived in that city.

I closed my practice in Bernalillo without much fanfare, and sold some equipment to one of my former residents who practiced in Albuquerque. It was a scramble to get to Fort Hood, as they wanted me to start on September thirtieth. I had to get my Advanced Cardiac Life Support (ACLS) certification; a requirement for the position. All local ACLS courses were full in the Albuquerque area, but I was able to locate a nurse from the University of New Mexico who was willing to come to my office in Bernalillo and teach me one-on-one. Staffcare paid her fees.

I had several phone conversations with Captain John Clay, acting Chief of Podiatry at Fort Hood. Apparently, he was told by his organization that he could pick and choose the one for this position. Staffcare told him they had chosen me already. This misunderstanding created some conflict initially between Dr. Clay and me who finally agreed to have me report for duty. Unfortunately, our first telephone encounters set the tone for some further conflict with John after I began working at the Darnall Army Community Hospital Podiatry Clinic at Fort Hood (name changed to Ft. Cavazos, since John Bell Hood was a Confederate officer during the Civil War).

In September I flew from Albuquerque to the Killeen/Fort Hood Regional Airport via Dallas, and rented a car. Linda stayed behind in Bernalillo and I lived in several motels in Killeen for three weeks. Unlike AAA, which uses their well-known black and red diamond ratings, I rate hotels and motels in the following EFM categories: fleabag, budget, better, and best. I've stayed in all types over the years. (We were once flea-bitten in a motel in Moab, Utah)

Staffcare only paid for me to stay in budget properties until I could find permanent housing.

Killeen has expanded and grown rapidly from its original downtown location outside the gates of Fort Hood. Most of the new businesses and motels are along the Route 190 corridor. Killeen was a company town, with the company being the United States Army. Most of the businesses and clubs catered to the young soldiers and their families. Fort Hood was considered to be the largest military base in the free world, with forty-five thousand active duty soldiers. There was a poster above the entrance to the Killeen Walmart that read,

"Fort Hood, Texas, Home of America's Hammer!!!"

Displayed on the poster was an outline of Texas with the unit crests of all the Army units stationed at Fort Hood. I took a photo of the sign and framed it.

I really am a patriot.

One of my colleagues characterized the antics of teenaged soldiers as similar to early college years of drinking, carousing and partying. I spent my first night at a budget property reserved for me by Staffcare. After suffering through a sleepless night due to the partying of young soldiers, I moved to another location. The next place was cockroach infested (definitely fleabag quality), and had its share of unsavory tenants.

I felt unsafe and unclean there.

I went back to the original place, and moved again from there to another place. I decided to keep my big suitcase in the rental car to make my frequent moves easier. I asked my contact at Staffcare if they would pay for me to stay at a better property. He said,

"I'm sorry, that's not in the budget."

I moved several more times due to traffic noise and more partying until I flew back to New Mexico to get the family.

Through a local rental agency in Albuquerque, Linda was able to find a tenant to rent our home. He was a physician beginning a new job at Presbyterian Hospital in Albuquerque.

He also turned out to be a slob.

I reported to Darnall Army Community Hospital early on my first morning. Staffcare's instructions were incomplete, and after finding the hospital AOD (Administrative Officer of the Day; a job I disliked when I was on active duty), I finally located the building where I needed to be. I began the in-processing procedures at Fort Hood while on Staffcare's payroll. The government in general, and the Army in particular, are quite inefficient when orienting new employees to their system. I went from one mindless required meeting to another before ever seeing my first patient, but at least I was being paid at my hourly rate.

I met the Chief of Surgery who almost welcomed me with a hug. He was a kind, gracious man who was a career Army surgeon. He said, "Thank you so much for coming to Darnall. Our podiatry clinic is very busy, and we really need your help."

Rumor was that he had been selected for promotion to Brigadier General, but declined the honor, as that would have taken him away from direct patient care. After getting to know him, I have no doubt that this rumor was true.

I did not have my own office or computer at first, so I shared a computer and desk with one of the podiatry nurses. She was a typical Texas gal who liked to over-organize events for the clinic. She insisted on having Hanukkah decorations as well as Christmas decorations at our holiday party. She did this out of respect for my Jewish colleague, Dr. Howard Richards and me.

I had no contact with the Army since I left Fort Meade, Maryland in 1982. Twenty-two -years later, very little had changed. Podiatrists were still assigned to the Medical Service Corps, but were exempt from AOD duty. They were still not receiving Professional Pay, as were the Army physicians. The Specialist five enlisted rank was eliminated, and a new Chief Warrant Officer Five rank was added. Other than technological changes corresponding to the times, the Army seemed very much the same as I remembered it. During the time I was at Fort Hood, the Army was in the process of phasing out the desert camouflage uniform for the pixilated uniform. Since we were at war, all soldiers wore these fatigues. I saw few soldiers in Class A uniforms and those were mostly recruiters.

I remembered enough about the Army to make a point to befriend the NCOIC (Non-Commissioned Officer-in-Charge) of the Podiatry Clinic. Staff Sergeant Raymond was the typical Army goldbrick and slacker. He reminded me of the cartoon character, Mort Walker's Sergeant Snorkel. He was a master at manipulating the system to avoid work, including faking medical conditions. Staff Sergeant Raymond was having a difficult time making the next rank of E-7, Sergeant First Class, and was faced with a possible "up or out" situation before he could retire at twenty years. He was not the sharpest knife in the drawer, but nevertheless I needed him to be an ally. He took me to the PX (Post Exchange) and I bought him lunch. The PX was disappointing from what I remembered it being at Fort Meade. It seemed like a Walmart without the sales tax.

Captain (Dr.) John Clay was the acting OIC (Officer-in-Charge) of the Podiatry Clinic. Major (Dr.) William Redman, the actual OIC was deployed to Iraq. Their plan was for John and Bill to split a one-year deployment, since Bill had already been there for a year's deployment and John had yet to go. I was hired to fill in for them for the year they were gone. Dr. Howard Richards was the other civilian podiatrist who had been working there for the past seven years. He was working under yearlong renewable contracts from an agency different from Staffcare. Howard was well liked by all, and rightfully so. We got along well from the start. Howard had sold his high-powered practice in Houston to move to the country with his wife. She was a nurse in the OR at Darnall and we worked together.

The Richards lived on a farm in San Saba (the actor Tommy Lee Jones was born there), which was seventy miles one way from Fort Hood. There they had acreage, a pool, horses, and raised bull mastiff dogs.

Howard also raised chickens and often brought freshly laid eggs into the clinic for people to take home. We had a refrigerator in the clinic for lunches and fresh eggs. I've never tasted better eggs than fresh laid. Howard had worked out a schedule of four ten-hour days with Fridays off.

Darnall Army Community Hospital recently became the C.R. Darnall Army Medical Center. The hospital had been staffed with many contractors in all departments such as Howard and me. After I left, the current Hospital Commander decided to eliminate as many contracts as possible and converted those into permanent government jobs. Howard was fortunate to have his contracting job converted to permanent employment, complete with all the government benefits we lacked as contractors. Unfortunately for him, he had to work five days a week after the change.

The change of designation from Community Hospital to Army Medical Center was well deserved. Rumor has it that retired generals living in San Antonio did not want to have Darnall compete with their local Brooke Army Medical Center for funding, so this upgrade for Darnall was long in coming. More babies were born at Fort Hood than anywhere else in the Army.

The hospital's namesake, Brigadier General Carl Rogers Darnall was an Army doctor who invented chlorination of water to sanitize municipal water supplies. The Fort Hood MEDDAC (Medical Department Activity) Unit Crest shows two opposing flasks of green chlorine gas superimposed with the medical serpent symbol to commemorate this milestone discovery in public health. Colonel John Bell Hood was in the Confederate Army, and Killeen/Fort Hood is located in his namesake Bell County.

The Podiatry Clinic staff also included two clerks. Our LPN (LVN in Texas) was Terry Valentino. Terry was from south of Rochester, New York, my hometown. Needless to say, we had much in common. Terry and his wife, a social worker at the hospital, moved to the area to be near their kids. Terry's job was to assist the podiatrists during surgery and to assist in clinic when not in the OR. Each of us had one day a week assigned in the OR, where we could schedule three or four cases per day. Terry was the best and most organized surgical assistant I had ever worked with. I trusted his judgment implicitly. I have no doubt that he could have easily performed many of the podiatric cases by himself if he had to, licensing and credentialing issues aside. Regarding his living in Texas, Terry often said, "If you weren't born in Texas and have no job here, you don't belong here."

He was right.

We became a close-knit group which I labeled "The pod squad," and often ate lunch together in the hospital cafeteria.

After working there about two months, the Surgery Department Administrator told me, "Dr. Meltzer, I advise you to start looking for another job.

I was taken off guard by her comment. "Why is that?"

"Once Captain Clay and Major Redman return from Iraq, your job here is done."

Of course, this was not what I was told by Staffcare. My contact at Staffcare lied to me to get me to accept the job. Fort Hood paid Staffcare a large fee on top of my salary, which explains their unethical recruiting technique at my expense. We had bought a house in Harker Heights with the expectation of my working there long-term. After I recovered from the initial shock of the reality of my temporary situation, I realized that the Administrator really did me a big favor. It took me the next nine months to find a permanent government job.

John Clay was a well-trained, self-assured podiatrist. He did his three-year residency in foot and ankle surgery at Fort Bragg, North Carolina. He was routinely performing major reconstructive cases on a weekly basis, and I learned from him. He also learned a few things from me. Of course, no one wanted to go to Iraq, and John was no exception. As a good Mormon, he and his wife had five children all under the age of eight. As the date of John's deployment got closer, he decided to pass off the majority of his postoperative patients to me. His patients were not happy about that. Even so, he enjoyed surgery so much that he did a case a few days before actually leaving for Iraq. I call that, "The cut and run policy."

I do not believe in treating patients like that.

John and I had differing philosophies regarding postoperative care. A few of his patients complained to him about my treatment as differing from his. He confronted me about this, and we agreed to disagree. He was young, bordering upon arrogant, and he was my acting boss. He went to the Surgery Administrator with his concerns. Perhaps this was one of those sentinel events in life. Linda and I did not enjoy living in Central Texas, and we would have missed out on the Montana experience had I been asked to stay at Fort Hood.

John and I eventually worked out our differences, and he paid me the ultimate compliment one surgeon can give to another, as he once said during a case he was assisting me with, "Evan, you have good hands."

I assisted him on a number of cases I had not done before, and I showed him my endoscopic plantar fasciotomy (cutting the ligament on the bottom of the foot using an arthroscope and a special small surgical blade to relieve chronic plantar fasciitis)and other procedures. He helped me with a Lisfranc's surgery (for a foot dislocation) and an external fixation case for a delayed union of a first metatarsal.

Howard, a capable surgeon in his own right also assisted me on some ankle and flatfoot cases. John had plans to leave the Army at the end of his commitment. Just to be safe, however, he applied for an Army Fellowship in advanced surgery. That program would have added to his committed time and probably have made him a career officer.

During my intensive job search, I came upon an opening for a job in Utah. I mentioned this to John. Mormon; Utah: a match made in heaven!

John ended up practicing in that multidisciplinary clinic in Utah after his Army discharge, thanks in part to me. Unfortunately, soon after entering private practice in Utah, John died of a brain tumor.

A clause in my contract allowed extra pay for taking call at the hospital. Howard, John and I informally divided the evening and weekend call schedule. Howard never had to come on weekends because he lived so far away. Soldiers injured or wounded in Iraq were stabilized there, and transferred to the large Army hospital in Landstuhl, Germany. From Germany, soldiers were then transferred to their home duty stations for definitive care. I took call on several occasions, including being called in to treat an injured soldier on Christmas Eve. I found this to be an extremely rewarding and gratifying experience.

On the personal front, Linda was in Bernalillo for the first few weeks of my arrival at Fort Hood while I worked during the day at Darnall. On weekends and evenings, I searched for a suitable home for our three dogs and us. Staffcare was paying for lodging and our initial efforts were spent in trying to find a rental house that would allow three dogs. I had the daunting task of trying to find a place that allowed three dogs, was mainly on one floor, that was new and in a good neighborhood. I finally located just such a house on Yak Trail in the Killeen suburb of Harker Heights. This was a rental property in excellent condition, but was managed by a shady rental agency often found near major military installations. Rental companies in the Killeen area had the policy of loaning out the keys to perspective tenants for their various vacant rental properties. The keys just had to be returned before close of business that day. I know that if I had a rental home listed with those agencies, I would not have wanted my keys loaned out to just anyone.

Staffcare tried to negotiate a fair rental for the Yak Trail house, but they could not reach an agreement with this sleazy company. Staffcare had a maximum limit they could spend on my housing, but they would not tell me exactly what it was. I toured many unsuitable properties, and was growing frustrated with the process. Finally, Linda suggested that I start looking at new homes to purchase, since she reasoned Staffcare was paying for the cost and they might as well pay for our mortgage. We expected to stay for years. I finally located a new home on Elk Trail, just a block from the home on Yak.

The builder had originally built the house as a rental, but he was asking far more for rent than Staffcare allowed. The house met most of Linda's requirements: new, all on one floor, a fenced in yard for the dogs, and the possibility of a doggy door, all in a good neighborhood. The front yard had one hundred fifty-year-old beautiful live oak trees, but the back yard was narrow, with three terraced areas supported by railroad timbers. I thought this area would be a great blank canvas for Linda to perform her usual landscaping magic.

Again, since Staffcare was paying the housing costs, I did not want to put much money of our own as a down payment. The builder had a cozy arrangement with a mortgage company in Austin, so I agreed to an eighty percent first mortgage with a twenty percent second mortgage. For a thousand dollars earnest money, I signed the agreement to purchase the house. This was the same sort of deal that had contributed to the housing and foreclosure crisis of 2008. For a thousand-dollars down payment I bought a three-hundred-thousand-dollar house with two mortgages. If you paid attention to this narrative, you realize Linda never saw this home. I usually had USAA as my insurance company, but for some reason decided to go with a local Texas bank for the homeowner's policy on the new home.

I flew back to Albuquerque for the annual balloon fiesta for the first weekend in October. For Linda's birthday in August, I bought a plane ticket for her lifelong friend, Jeanne Danboise, to visit us. She came for the balloon fiesta and practically melted her camera taking photos. We arranged for the move at our expense of our household goods from Bernalillo to Harker Heights. I flew back to New Mexico the following week to drive Linda and the dogs to Texas. As we drove up to our new house, upon seeing it, Linda cried. "Don't ever buy a house without your spouse first seeing it!"

Our household goods arrived without much damage, and we began the settling in process. The builder installed a doggy door to the back patio. Linda soon met Cindy Tuttle while walking the dogs one day. Bob Tuttle was a Colonel, and the family was living in a rental house down Elk Trail. Cindy and Linda became friends, and soon we began socializing with them as couples. Bob injured his foot in Iraq, soon after his deployment. He was sent to Landstuhl, Germany, for surgery. He had a Lisfranc's injury that was surgically repaired there. His deployment was cut short, and he returned to his duty station at Fort Hood. He was also a patient in our clinic.

Bob was the chief financial officer of all Army units stationed at Fort Hood. He was in charge of purchasing and procuring all equipment needed to maintain forty-five thousand soldiers during war time. Bob and Cindy were a nice couple with a teenage boy and girl. Bob was weighing his options regarding retirement at the time we met. The Tuttles had lived all around Europe and the States, and had never owned their own home before. They were building a vacation home in South Carolina at the beach.

Just before Christmas, Linda called me at work one morning. She had noticed a foul stench coming from the laundry drain some days prior and now was finding raw sewage seeping into the bathtubs and onto the floors. I immediately called my new insurance agent at the bank for guidance. He told me to call a certain environmental cleanup company, as the sewage was obviously contaminated and unsafe. He assured me that all this was covered under my policy.

When I got home that evening, I found this company from Waco in the process of ripping up our brand-new laminate flooring, the sheet rock walls and insulation down to the studs in the master bedroom, living room, and dining room. They sprayed disinfectant on the concrete slab and left several large fans on to dry out the house. Before leaving that night, they demanded a thousand-dollar check as a down payment on the work they had done.

The Tuttles stopped by that evening, and were shocked at what they saw. They offered to have us stay with them, but fortunately one half of the house was not affected. The bank's insurance agent also said all temporary housing expenses would be covered if we needed to stay in a motel until repairs were completed. Fortunately, we elected to sleep in the undamaged half of the house. Naturally we called our builder, who immediately denied any responsibility for the problem. He even alluded to the fact that we probably caused the problem by flushing a Pamper or similar item down the toilet.

We have no small children and had a long history of home ownership and responsible toilet use.

The builder did call his plumber who snaked a video camera down the sewer line. They found a soda can lodged in the pipe, located under the pavement of Elk Trail in front of the house. Further inspection of the line also revealed a crushed sewer line beyond the soda can directly under the road. Neighbors told us that while the house was being built, kids used to swing from our oak trees and that they might have thrown a soda can down an open pipe.

It now seemed as if the town of Harker Heights had the major responsibility for this disaster.

When George W. Bush was governor of Texas, he supported a business and municipality- friendly environment. He also limited medical malpractice claims to a maximum of two hundred-fifty-thousand dollars. Even though property taxes in Texas were obscenely high, apparently municipalities like Harker Heights were not responsible for maintaining a properly functioning sewer system. We soon learned that our insurance did not cover any of the damage we incurred and that our insurance agent had misled us. The environmental cleanup of our home cost in excess of four-thousand dollars. It cost us about another twelve-thousand-dollars to repair the damage.

We met with the City Manager of Harker Heights who basically denied any responsibility for our damage. We finally hired an attorney, but had to drive sixty miles to Waco to find an impartial lawyer. We threatened our builder with a lawsuit. He paid us for our repairs and Harker Heights agreed to pay us the four-thousand plus for the cleanup, all without admitting any fault on their part. The City excavated a fifteen-foot deep trench in the road in front of our house to repair the crushed pipe. We later found several places where the City had done the same repair in the neighborhood and heard that our next-door neighbor had a similar sewer backup problem. I thought it interesting that if the City did not admit fault, why did they somehow find the need to dig up the road and make the required sewer repairs? They also installed a water cutoff valve in our front yard at no expense to us.

Our builder said he would attempt to sue Harker Heights to recover his losses. Ultimately, the original developer of the Country Trails subdivision was responsible, but he was a "good ol' boy," and would escape all this unharmed. I immediately dropped the existing insurance policy and switched back to USAA. Of course, USAA would not allow me to purchase the forty-dollar-per-year rider for sewer backup on that property. As a non-native living in Texas, I felt totally defenseless when dealing with the local government and municipality of Harker Heights.

Terry Valentino was right again.

My contract paid me on a strictly hourly basis, and did not allow for paid vacation. In February, Linda and I decided to take a few days off to go to South Padre Island. This was a popular destination for college students for spring break, but we were going during the off-season.

We stayed at the dog-friendly LaQuinta right on the beach. The dogs loved running on the sand and chasing seabirds. There was a large crowd of "snowbirds" (like sea birds without feathers) from Wisconsin and Minnesota who always stayed there the same time each winter for a month. We fit right in. At five o'clock, the hotel served complimentary beer, wine and snacks. We had a wonderful time.

My mother's health had been declining for several years. She and dad visited us in New Mexico and her poor health was quite apparent then. She was diagnosed with a particularly virulent form of dementia called Dementia with Lewy Bodies. This unfortunate illness is characterized with Parkinson-like symptoms, including loss of balance, and delusional behavior. Mom had gained quite a bit of weight recently and had taken some bad falls. Dad had great difficulty picking her up, as he had his own health problems. I had plans to fly to Philadelphia on Friday after we returned from South Padre. Mom was in the hospital and my sister called to say, "Mom was not doing well."

Mom died on Thursday night, before I was leaving the next day. I took the next week off for the funeral and religious services at my sister's house. Linda stayed in Texas to watch the dogs.

Mom and Dad were married for sixty-one years, and Dad was devastated. They had a secret code between them that Dad had engraved on a charm for Mom's gold bracelet when I was still a child.

On it was engraved the letters, YLHFE, "Your loving husband forever."

That charm was located right next to the one with her mother's Eagle pin, given to her by my Boy Scout troop in honor of my becoming an Eagle Scout.

Forever had finally arrived.

Dad asked me, "Do you want to see Mom?"

"Yes, please take me to the funeral home."

I took the elevator to the basement alone to view Mom's body. I did not recognize her.

It was a very emotional but necessary task.

I stayed with Dad the week I was there, but he hardly spoke. During Mom's illness, there was a lady her age who befriended them. She was the mother of one of my sister's friends. Arlene assisted Mom and Dad until Mom's death. I did not realize that during that time Dad and Arlene became close. Arlene, a widow, was an educated woman who was an accomplished musician, actor, artist, and community volunteer. Dad was a painter, so they had much in common.

Within a few months of Mom's death, Dad and Arlene became a couple. My sister Sherry and I moved Dad into an upscale senior living center a mile from Sherry's house, and I learned later it was located a floor above Arlene's apartment.

I had met Arlene during Mom's funeral and she seemed pleasant. It took me some time to get used to Dad's seeing her after spending so much of his life with Mom. Dad would later say, "If it weren't for her, I'd be dead by now."

How could I take exception with that statement?

By August, I had not heard anything from the Billings Area (administrative headquarters for Browning) regarding the job I had applied for with the Indian Health Service and began to get nervous about future employment. I had obtained my Texas podiatry license, but two private practice opportunities there did not pan out.

I was also tripped up for a local VA job just twenty minutes from Harker Heights by my old nemesis, IS. My neighbor was Chief of Orthopedics at the Temple, Texas VA. A former fellow New Yorker from Brooklyn, he had been living in Texas for many years and had started another young family. He was also a Colonel in the Army Reserves, and we worked together at Fort Hood while he was on his Active Duty for Training. He was also my patient. Early one morning, he came bounding into my office at Darnall with exciting news.

"Evan, Tom Douglas told me he is leaving the Temple VA for a two year leave of absence." Dr. Douglas was Chief of Podiatry. The Colonel said,

"If you get the job, we could carpool to work together. Of course, I can't guarantee you'll get the job. But I'll do what I can to help."

Linda and I were not exactly enamored with the Killeen area, but we owned a house there, and it seemed like the answer for us at the time. It would at least give us entry back into the government system with all the coveted benefits we were looking for.

The Acting Chief of Podiatry at the Temple VA happened to be making some networking phone calls to other VA's around the country looking for promising applicants for the soon to be vacant position. Unfortunately for me, one of those calls was to IS in Albuquerque. After that phone call, I spoke by phone with Dan, the acting podiatry chief at the Temple VA who was quite gracious. He said, "I tend to disregard one bad recommendation if I hear several other good ones. I realize this just might be a personality clash."

My neighbor was not so forgiving.

Soon after my phone call with Dan, I ran into my neighbor. He said, "Dan called me about his conversation with your old chief in Albuquerque."

I asked him, "What did Dan say?"

The Colonel said, "Dan said that he was not complimentary."

I replied, "He fabricated false information so he could get rid of me."

My neighbor said, "I was not happy to hear those criticisms about you."

"Colonel, you know me and worked with me. Don't you consider what you personally experience first hand as more trustworthy than what you hear third hand?"

He said, "I believe what Dan tells me."

I replied, "That speaks volumes about your true character."

I left in a huff.

I lost respect for that orthopedist and neighbor who did not even have the decency to credit the collegial time we spent together at Darnall as ample evidence against the falsehoods spread by IS, not to mention my successful treatment of his foot and ankle problem. I realized that my behavior with my neighbor was not very dignified, but I was angry about the position he took. I applied for the VA job in Temple, but withdrew my application upon accepting the job in Browning. I guess I did not wish to face the possible rejection of my application. I saw my neighbor periodically around the neighborhood, before and after going to Browning, but our encounters were always perfunctory and superficial. Linda believed he was truly surprised when she told him the Jackson VA had hired me.

I hired the same attorney in Albuquerque I had used for my previous VA issues to deal with IS's most recent character assassination attempt. At my request, the lawyer wrote a letter, copying the VA Director, Chief of Staff, and IS's immediate boss, the new Chief of Surgical Service. I could not afford nor tolerate any more unfounded allegations regarding my professional abilities, as I was actively seeking re-employment in the government. I had recently visited with several of my former residents from the Albuquerque VA at a professional meeting. It seems the new surgery chief had not been at all pleased with IS. In fact, the new chief demoted him from Chief of Podiatry, replacing him with the same doctor from Fort Bragg who helped train Dr. Clay. As IS often used to say (about others), "He was a legend in his own mind."

There was no better expression to describe IS. He no longer works at the VA as he was forced to resign due to allegations of sexual harassment of a VA nurse. (After retiring and registering as a veteran patient at the Albuquerque VA, I also learned that Steve Frank had been fired. He had a construction company that took too much of his time away from his duties at the VA). As my mother used to say, "What goes around comes around."

* * *

August 27th is Linda's birthday and she wanted to celebrate at the Johnson Ranch. It also happens to be the birthday of former President Lyndon B. Johnson. Johnson's Western Whitehouse was located near Fredericksburg, Texas, a scenic drive from Fort Hood through the Texas hill country. The President is buried in the family plot within sight of the house. Every August 27th, the Johnson family holds a birthday celebration on the ranch, which was open to the public. They served Texas watermelon, birthday cake, and cookies to all visitors on that day. As we were walking around the property, Linda spied a woman in a wheelchair being pushed by a younger woman. Tourists were milling about the couple paying no attention to them. Linda said to me, "Isn't that Ladybird Johnson?"

We walked up to the two women and I said, "Excuse me, but aren't you the Johnsons?'

"We're the Meltzers visiting from Fort Hood." The younger woman extended her hand and said, "Hi, I'm Lucy Baines Johnson and I am pleased to meet you. I'm glad you're here to help celebrate daddy's birthday."

Ms. Johnson asked me, "What do you do at Fort Hood?"

I replied, "I'm a doctor there."

"How do you enjoy treating our soldiers at Fort Hood?"

I replied, "I feel honored and privileged to be able to do so."

Ms. Johnson then turned around to the woman in the wheelchair and said in a very polished and strong voice, "Mother, these are the Meltzers who are visiting from Fort Hood. Dr. Meltzer takes care of our soldiers."

Ladybird had suffered a stroke and could not walk or talk, but her eyes lit up and she smiled as Linda and I took turns shaking her hand. Both women seemed pleased to be recognized. Unfortunately, I did not have my camera to record that historic event.

We soon noticed an athletic looking young man in a red baseball cap and an earpiece standing nearby. He quickly decided we were no threat to the former First Lady and her daughter. Former presidents and their families are protected for life by the Secret Service. Ladybird was an environmental advocate as First Lady, and there was a spectacular wildflower garden bearing her name that we had previously visited near Austin.

Chapter Four

MONTANA, The Last Best Place.

2005-2007

My contract job at Darnall Army Community Hospital at Fort Hood was coming to a close. I really enjoyed treating soldiers. As an Army veteran and patriot myself, I felt that this group of brave individuals, including former soldiers (veterans) were the most deserving of all groups for free government medical care. Soldiers are the point of the spear; carrying out the policies of our lawmakers-whether they are right or wrong. I also enjoyed the practice mix itself, with healthy patients who would actually heal. I enjoyed the heavy emphasis on sports medicine and surgery that this group required. A soldier's mantra was, "Mine is not to reason why, mine is just to do or die."

The Army was good at presenting awards, and my brief service as a civilian was duly recognized. The department took me out to my favorite restaurant for an awards banquet. They presented me with a beautiful wood name plate for my desk, and a framed photo of Darnall Army Hospital signed by all my coworkers, much like my high school yearbook signed by my classmates. I was particularly touched by my boss Bill Redman's comments on the photo, which read in part, "It has been an honor to have you back at an Army Hospital."

It was an honor for me to serve again.

The Chief of Orthopedics presented me with a Department of the Army Certificate of Appreciation on behalf of the hospital Commander. It read:

For outstanding dedication in support of Global War on Terrorism as a Podiatric Foot Surgeon, Podiatry Clinic, Darnall Army Community Hospital, Fort Hood, Texas for the period 01 October 2004 thru September 2005. His motivation, selfless service, and dedication to duty are in keeping with the highest traditions of government service and reflect great credit upon him, the Podiatry Profession, and Darnall Army Community Hospital.

The hospital Commander was sent to the Pentagon soon after I left, and was promoted to Brigadier General. She was the highest-ranking psychiatrist in the Army, and worked on the pervasive problem of Post Traumatic Stress Disorder among our returning troops.

They also presented me with my official framed Army photo that was displayed in the clinic along with Howard, John and Bill's during my tenure.

These awards, along with the PA Preceptor of the Year award were prominently displayed on my office wall at the Jackson VA.

I was humbled by the whole experience.

I received more recognition in my one year at Fort Hood than I ever received for all my subsequent years at the VA.

In September 2005, Jonie Hind, MD, the Clinical Director of Blackfeet Community Hospital in Browning, Montana, called me. She asked me if I had ever been to Browning before. Some thirty plus years before, in another life, I traveled with my family to Glacier National Park. While I did not specifically remember Browning, I know I must have passed through there and may have even camped there outside the Park. After living there, I now know why she asked that question. While not formally allowed to offer me the job (that had to be done by the HR department in Billings), she not so subtly hinted I was on the top of her list. This same job had originally been posted on USAJOBS in February and I applied at that time. My application materials were mailed back to me in April with a note saying the posting had been canceled. The job was re-posted in June, and I re-applied. I later learned why this happened. A podiatrist who had worked in Browning earlier was trying to negotiate a package deal to return to Browning that also included employing his wife. The negotiations fell through, as the hospital did not have a position for her. That was why the job was re-posted.

I was now well-versed at navigating through the locum tenens websites for podiatry, and found a listing for a temporary job in Browning-the same place I had applied for permanent work. I applied and was immediately accepted. In fact, my Fort Hood job ended September thirtieth, and this agency wanted me to start in Browning on October third. It would have been close to impossible for me to drive the 1900 miles over that weekend to get there by then.

About a week after signing a contract with the locum tenens agency to work as a temp in Browning for only three to six months, I received the formal offer from Billings Area for the permanent position. I was in Howard Richard's truck driving with him to a graduation ceremony for graduating Army Physician Assistants I helped train when the formal call of the job offer came from Billings HR on my cell phone. I was preparing to deliver a speech to my graduating PA students and their families, and also to proudly receive their award to me for being the Fort Hood PA Preceptor of the Year.

Of course, I accepted the permanent job, but I thought I might have a contractual problem with the temp agency. This company turned out to be just a "mom and pop" agency located in Pennsylvania, specializing in mainly placing nurses for locum tenens positions. They were not pleasant to work with, and I hired an attorney to deal with them. My father lived near my sister in West Chester, PA, so I hired Dad's attorney who was practicing in PA. It turns out that the temp agency never sent me back a signed copy by them of the contract I signed, so my attorney advised me to withdraw my offer to be employed by them. The company threatened a lawsuit, and my lawyer asked them to put him in touch with their lawyer. I heard nothing further from them after that letter. Occasionally, lawyers are worth their fees.

After arriving on station in Browning, the Indian Health Service was still obligated to this Pennsylvania agency to provide a contract podiatrist, even though I was perfectly capable of handling the work load myself. They were unable to provide another podiatrist who could be successfully credentialed, and gave up after three doctors could not meet IHS credentialing standards.

I had agreed to work at the Blackfeet Hospital at the salary level GS-14 Step ten. This was the top salary being offered for podiatrists employed by the Indian Health Service at that time. After accepting the job and that salary, Dr. Hind asked, "Do you mind if I also offer you a twenty five percent recruitment bonus?"

"No, I certainly don't mind at all!"

I was able to get my start date moved to mid-October so I could comfortably make the trip from Harker Heights, Texas to Browning and arrange for the move of our household goods. They had been waiting for a podiatrist there for a year and a half, so a few extra days was not going to be a problem. Our plan was for Linda to drive up to Browning with me, and then fly back to Texas for the winter. After all, we had chosen the southwest and Texas largely because of Linda's health. Montana winters were not exactly what Linda bargained for. We figured we would somehow work this out, either by my getting another job in a warmer place, or by having a second home in a warm climate. Ironically, Linda and I had recently been discussing the possibility of owning a summer cabin in cool Montana after suffering through the hot, humid Texas summer.

We arrived in Browning without any lodging arrangements the week before I was to begin work. We located the hospital, and found Bob Jones who was in charge of housing. As a contractor, I was promised housing for the duration of my contract. I had been corresponding with Jones via email before our arrival regarding the various permanent housing that was available. We found Jones on the phone as we entered his office, who could not be bothered to acknowledge our presence until he finished his call- not a good sign. After he hung up the phone, I introduced myself and asked, "Do you have any temporary housing available until our permanent quarters are ready?"

He said, "I don't have very many".

"I only need one place. How about the one that was previously reserved for the contract podiatrist, which was supposed to be me?"

He showed us to a 1930s era single family shack down the hill from the hospital that Linda promptly renamed the "flop house". Our only other alternative was a run-down motel outside of

Browning. We took the flop house at eleven-fifty per day, clean linens and towels included. I later learned my friends referred to this place as the "crack house." The basement was filled with trash, a broken washer and dryer and the living area was filthy. I had not seen such squalid living conditions since I was in college. Bob Jones was the consummate government employee who can give you at least five reasons in great detail why something cannot be done. We have all encountered the camp counselor can-do type. Jonie Hind was one stellar example. Jones was the poster guy of the can't do type.

We cleaned the place as best we could, and emptied our stuff into the house. Linda took the squeaky double bed in the larger bedroom, and I took the bunk room. The wiring was so old I was afraid of fire every time I turned on a switch.

The next day we inspected quarters number twelve that was to be our permanent housing. Each set of government quarters was assigned to one of Jones' handymen. Ours was assigned to get number twelve ready before the moving truck arrived from Texas. His boss was Bob Jones. Local union rules for maintenance workers mandated a coffee break from 10-10:30, lunch from 12-1, and an afternoon break from 3-3:30. Our man would show up around nine, paint about two square feet of wall until the morning break. He would then drive his truck the one hundred yards back to the maintenance shop to visit with his coworkers over coffee.

We might see him next sometime after 1pm, where he might paint another two square feet, or maybe spend an hour cleaning a sink. Or we might see him again at nine the next morning. It seems he was always running out to get something he needed to work on number twelve. Home Depot and Lowe's were each two hours away.

It was quite clear to us that the carpets would not get shampooed before the movers arrived, and the carpets were filthy. A family of five had lived there for twelve years.

Linda and I were convinced that our presence at number twelve would have no influence whatsoever on the speed at which our guy would complete the renovation.

I said, "Let's go explore Whitefish."

We left Browning to explore the west side of the mountains prior to my starting work on Monday, October seventeenth. Whitefish charmed us. The town reminded Linda of Minoa, the railroad town east of Syracuse, New York where she grew up.

Whitefish is an upscale small town, with a lake and beach in the summer, and Big Mountain (now called Whitefish Mountain Resort) in the winter for skiing. The town is a major railroad hub for western Montana. We explored the Going-To-The-Sun Road and the Lake McDonald area of Glacier National Park. Linda had a one-way airline ticket from Calgary, Alberta Canada to Dallas and Killeen/Fort Hood on Sunday, so we drove to Calgary on Saturday. It was a sad weekend, because we knew we were beginning an indefinite geographic separation. The plan was for Linda to return to Browning in the spring of 2006 and spend the good weather months with me there.

Sunday morning came soon enough, and we tearfully parted company at the Calgary airport. I sadly drove the three-and-a-half hours back to the flop house, while Linda flew safely back to our home in Harker Heights, Texas. I began work on Monday, and met my new assistant, Karen Green. Karen had worked with my predecessor, a podiatrist with Indian Preference.

That doctor left Browning under somewhat mysterious circumstances and conflicting reports concerning his departure.

The Indian Health Service is the only U.S. government agency that is allowed to legally discriminate due to ethnic origin. This is what is referred to as Indian Preference. To receive that preferential title, one must prove their tribal ancestry and have this information verified. Job applicants with Indian Preference are given first consideration for jobs within IHS if all other qualifications are similar to non-preference candidates. In fact, one of my IHS podiatrist colleagues from Crow Agency whom I later met told me, "The primary purpose of the Indian Health Service is to provide jobs for Native Americans, and secondarily to provide health care."

While his remarks were meant to be sarcastic, as with any sarcasm, there is usually a load of truth behind them based on what I heard about my predecessor's exit from Browning.

Karen Green was a friend of my predecessor as well as being his assistant. They remained in contact well into my tenure at Browning. Karen was a Native originally from the Fort Peck Reservation in northeastern, Montana. She became my friend also, and proved invaluable at assisting me with sorting out all the family relations among the Blackfeet patients. Her husband Chuck was Blackfeet. The biggest favor Karen ever did for me soon after my arrival was to put the word out through the community grapevine that "Dr. Meltzer does not prescribe narcotics".

This information spread rapidly, and I was seldom bothered by drug seeking patients. Of course, I always prescribed narcotics for my post-op surgical patients, but Karen's announcement made my life much easier in that regard.

My immediate supervisor was the Clinical Director, Jonie Hind. Dr. Hind was without a doubt the best boss I ever had. Her answer to any question or request I had was always, "Yes".

She was the antithesis of Bob Jones. Jonie was a young woman with two small children and her husband, Richard. The week I began my job, I asked, "Would I be able to work a compressed work week?"

"What schedule did you have in mind?"

"How about four ten-hour days with Friday off?"

"How does four nine-hour days with four hours on Friday morning sound? We need you here every day," she said.

"Done deal," I replied

This schedule allowed Linda and me to take off for our trips the following summer as soon as I got home at noon on Friday. I was considered a Title Five employee. I didn't completely understand what that meant, except that I was required to keep accurate records of my work time. Every two weeks I had to turn in my time sheet to my timekeeper. As a professional, I hated clock watching. As a VA employee, I'd always worked until the last patient of the day was seen, finished my paper work and then gone home.

Under this system, I was obligated to stay at work until the clock said it was time to leave. Jonie even had a discussion with the medical staff regarding the installation of a time clock-which I (and they) found repugnant. The only advantage was that Title Five employees received either compensation time or overtime pay if they are called in after their normal duty hours. Another advantage occurred when attending a professional meeting on a weekend. All that time was comp or overtime. Nevertheless, I appreciated being a Title 38 employee at the VA, where I could leave when finished with my duties regardless of the time.

Jonie was a master at multitasking; very capable at balancing her various roles at work and with her family. She remained as Clinical Director until she left for private practice. Jonie was very happy in Browning, but an incident involving her husband, Richard changed all that. Richard was a graduate of the Ivy League,

University of Pennsylvania, and was a member of their Varsity wrestling team. He was a good student and top wrestler from Wyoming. He was awarded a full four-year wrestling scholarship to Penn.

Richard and Jonie were high school sweethearts. Richard was mostly a stay-at-home dad watching his young children while Jonie worked at the hospital. He had a part time job as the wrestling coach for Browning High School. In an attempt to motivate one of his talented high school wrestlers who was saddened by the death of a distant relative, the kid's father took offense at Richard's misunderstood remarks.

"I'm sorry to hear about the death of your cousin. You are a talented wrestler, and I believe you can take the state title in your weight class."

"Coach, I'm so broken up about my cousin's death I don't think I can do it."

"Sure you can, and I'll help as much as I can."

Richard was fired over that incident and the kid's dad threatened to kill Richard.

Browning never had such a strong wrestling program before Richard's tenure as coach. Needless to say, to protect her family Jonie made plans to leave Browning as soon as she could find a suitable job in private practice. After her departure, there was a huge void that could not be filled. No other physician desired the job, and it was eventually split between two reluctant doctors. Jim Blackweasel, the hospital CEO actually offered me the position, but I respectfully declined.

I did not want to relinquish my Friday afternoons and deal with all the headaches for the few thousand extra dollars a year. I also knew I would be leaving at some point in the future. Jonie joined a family practice in Cody, Wyoming nearer to hers and Richard's home town of Gillette. (Sadly, a few years later, Richard died in his sleep at age 37.)

Jonie returned for a week in June as a volunteer. She immediately picked up where she left off without missing a beat. At a staff meeting, one of the ER physicians asked,

"When are you coming back to work?"

It was great to see her again.

I had worked at several Indian Health centers while in private practice in New Mexico. Every tribe or Pueblo had its own cultural idiosyncrasies. The Cochiti Tribe of New Mexico would not show up for their scheduled appointments on Bread Baking Day. The Blackfeet Tribe was not much different. Like other Native Americans I had treated, they were not a healthy group. Diabetes and obesity were very common problems, along with the corresponding conditions of heart disease and hypertension. Drug and alcohol addiction were also major problems and frequent causes of horrible fatal motor vehicle accidents. Dental health was also poor, even though care was available to every enrolled tribal member.

My late friend Harold once asked me, "Evan, do you know what the worst drug is on the reservation?"

"Sure, it's narcotics."

"Nope, it's sugar," said Harold.

It was commonplace to see toddlers drinking Coke or other soft drinks directly from baby bottles or sippy cups. Visiting pediatric dentists were kept busy extracting rotten teeth from very young children.

The Blackfeet have a strong entitlement attitude, and many did not appreciate the quality and quantity of free medical care they received. I had a difficult time dealing with noncompliance issues among my patients. During my nineteen years of private practice in Ithaca, I do not recall a single patient who failed to show up for a scheduled postoperative appointment. That was such a prevalent problem in Browning that I stopped performing elective foot surgery for my last six months there. I also drafted a special consent form, outlining the schedule of postoperative appointments, and the reasons for each one. If the patients refused to sign this form, I would not schedule their non-emergent surgery. The general "no-show" rate in Browning was at times above forty percent. Patients with limb threatening conditions would not keep their appointments for what I considered trivial reasons.

"I was shopping in Great Falls", or

"I had to attend my second cousin's once removed funeral".

My sage wife once told me, "Evan, you can't save people from themselves".

On one of my flights to Texas to visit Linda, I sat next to a financial advisor from Denver. We struck up a conversation, and he asked me,

"What line of work are you in?"

"I'm a doctor with the Indian Health Service."

"That is an honorable thing to do," he said.

I realize that a significant part of my life has been geared towards service to others. My first professional job was teaching, but as I wrote earlier, the pay was so little I struggled to provide for my family. I was never greedy, as I consider greed one of the worst vices. While in private practice in Ithaca, New York my goal was to provide a comfortable lifestyle for my family and be able to invest the maximum allowable towards retirement. I was never interested in flashy consumerism. Public service had provided similar professional and financial rewards without the headaches of running a private solo medical practice.

Regions of the country define medical care in the United States: urban, suburban, rural, and frontier. Only Montana and Wyoming had the distinction of having the "frontier" label. I am not certain exactly what defines these regions, but it was related to distances from specialty medical care and services. There are some medical services not available anywhere in the state of Montana, and our hospital would often fly critical patients to Seattle. Those who practice medicine and surgery in a frontier setting often are required to go beyond what another provider would normally do in an urban or other environment.

I was impressed with each of the family doctors, and would have felt confident if I were their patient. There were six family physicians at Blackfeet Community Hospital; Jonie Hind was there for my first year. In addition to their clinical responsibilities as family doctors, each was required to work in the Emergency Department. Every weekend, one of these doctors was on call to the inpatients. Except for one, all had OB/GYN privileges and delivered babies. We also had one full time OB/GYN physician and at least one contracted OB/GYN physician available twenty-four/seven for cesarean sections and other high-risk patients. One of the senior family doctors was Chief of Surgery, which is an interesting title for a family doctor. He had assisted a previous general surgeon on gall bladder surgeries, and had a considerable amount of on-the-job training.

I was appointed Chairman of the Surgical Committee that dealt with policies regarding delivery of surgical care at the hospital. I was the only true surgical specialist on staff at the time. The committee met monthly, and I always emailed an agenda to each member a week ahead of the meetings. Dr. Hind, the Clinical

Director and my boss for my first year always managed to have timely topics to add to the agenda. She made my job as committee chairman considerably easier. A seventy-two-year old general surgeon from Maui, Hawaii and Durango, Colorado joined the staff in the spring before I left.

Prior to his arrival, we had contract general surgeons from Great Falls who would perform routine general cases such as gall bladder removals and hernia repairs. The new doctor was a physically fit, capable surgeon who did not want to retire. He worked four weeks on, and two weeks off. He was on call twenty-four/seven during his four weeks on, and then he would go back to his home in Durango for the two weeks. The Great Falls or Kalispell surgical group would cover for him during his two weeks off. The surgeon took over my locker in the operating room, and of course became Chairman of the Surgical Committee when I left. I was not sure if he also took over the title of Chief of Surgery.

One of my other assigned duties was to visit a remote clinic twenty-eight miles south of Browning, in a place called Heart Butte. Heart Butte Clinic was built to serve the small population of Blackfeet who lived in or near that community. The physical plant of the clinic was relatively new and of pleasing architecture. A family physician and nurse staffed the Clinic on Monday, Tuesday, Thursday and Friday. A fully-equipped dental clinic was also on site. The facility included a small pharmacy and blood draw lab. All staff rotated from Blackfeet Hospital.

My job description included providing podiatry services there once a month. Karen Green would coordinate my schedule, and she and I would sign out a GSA government vehicle and make the monthly drive. We had to bring our basic podiatry instruments along with us just like I had to do working at remote clinics in New Mexico. The Heart Butte Clinic had no x-ray facilities, so any patient requiring that service would have to make the trip to

Browning. While it was above my pay grade to question why the Clinic even existed, I believed it would have been more cost effective to close it and provide daily transportation for patients to and from Browning to access services at the main hospital. Personal transportation was a problem for many of the indigent Blackfeet.

The Heart Butte Clinic Administrator was the former Head Nurse at the Hospital. Before I arrived in Browning, James Blackweasel, the Hospital CEO, exiled her to that post for alleged poor performance. The replacement Head Nurse was a very competent professional. For some reason, the Clinic Administrator (CA) took an immediate dislike to me. I soon discovered she had some unpleasant experiences with one of my predecessors, and branded all of us podiatrists as problems. The CA would travel to Browning on Wednesday to take care of administrative matters, and stirred up trouble for me on several occasions.

I asked my boss, Dr. Jonie Hind to conduct a meeting to attempt to work out our differences. The CA agreed to work together with me, but our professional relationship remained strained after that meeting. The only patient complaint I ever received during my time at the Blackfeet reservation came from an old woman from Heart Butte. I have no doubt that the CA assisted her in drafting that letter.

The drive from Browning to Heart Butte was beautiful but dangerous. The Heart Butte Road was a secondary paved road with many twists and turns, and a hazardous steep grade approaching a bridge over the Two Medicine River. During the winter, the drive was particularly treacherous. There were numerous fatal crashes on that road, compounded by alcohol, weather, geography, and poor vehicle maintenance. GSA vehicles are basic Detroit models, and the maintenance staff to drive back and forth to their coffee breaks commandeered the four-wheel drive vehicles.

Driving south from Browning along the treeless high plains, the mountains of the Bob Marshall and Great Bear Wilderness Areas to the west provided a sweeping panorama into pristine country. One regret I had is not having trekked into the "Bob", as it is called by locals. I was told it takes at least a week on horseback to travel in and out of that wild place.

The Wilderness Act of 1964 set aside millions of acres of forever wild lands, mostly in the western U.S. Many western ranchers, farmers and miners have opposed the creation of new wilderness areas, claiming that these lands are saved for the enjoyment of the few elite liberals from both coasts. These are roadless areas that are only accessible on foot, horseback or man-powered boats (canoes or kayaks). No mining, logging, drilling or ranching is permitted. I am a staunch supporter of Wilderness, and have had some uncomfortable discussions with my native Montana friend, Harold regarding this sensitive subject.

James Blackweasel was the CEO of the hospital. Jim is a Blackfeet tribal member who graduated from Northern Montana University in Havre, where he played basketball and studied to become a school teacher. He previously had several tribal jobs, and was finally hired by the Blackfeet Tribe to run the hospital. Jim was very much a hands-on leader, who was often seen roaming around the hospital picking up trash with his gloved hands.

Every Monday, Wednesday and Friday mornings the medical staff had patient rounds in the conference room. Their attending physician presented every inpatient to the medical staff. Jim attended every meeting.

Unfortunately, Jim ran the hospital as if he personally owned it. In my opinion, he did not possess the skill-set to direct a federal medical facility. While on one hand admitting a lack of medical knowledge, he often inappropriately intervened in some medical scenarios. One of the emergency room nurses actually threw him out of the ER for looking at a medical chart of a patient, stating that was none of his business. He sent another nurse who was having personality conflicts with the head nurse in the OR to the Crow Agency for six months. That nurse received a glowing report about her performance at Crow.

I initially gained Jim's respect as he attended my Surgical Committee meetings. He was also my patient. After Jonie Hind left, Jim asked me if I would consider the Clinical Director's job. I was honored by the request, but respectfully declined.

One morning I drove Jim and Tim Makes Cold Weather to Cut Bank to meet with the administrator of their hospital. Tim was the assistant CEO and also my neighbor. We discussed recruiting a general surgeon we could share with her hospital and ours. Jim treated Tim and me to lunch at a café in Cut Bank after the meeting. I continued to have good relations with Jim until I notified him of my pending job in Jackson.

After returning from my site visit to Jackson, I knew I had the job offer. I was in a quandary as to how and when to announce my transfer, since my actual start date in Jackson was yet undetermined and dependent on so many factors. I consulted with my assigned HR person in Jackson who told me that as a federal employee, I could not be fired for transferring to another government agency. Apparently, Jim Blackweasel did not know that. During a phone conversation with the HR Department in Jackson, the official advised me, "Since Jackson will be contacting your employer shortly, and you should let them know sooner rather than later about you're pending transfer."

Jim Blackweasel knew about my personal situation and he got to know Linda when she was there. I asked him into my office and said, "Jim, I've accepted a job at the Jackson, Mississippi VA hospital." At first, he seemed thoughtful and understanding.

"When does the new job start?"

"They are aiming for the day after Labor Day, but we both know about government paperwork."

"Dr. Meltzer, I understand you want to be reunited with your wife. I know she's not too fond of Browning."

"Jim, the animal cruelty and other factors really affected her. As I drove her out of Browning for Texas, she said she would never set foot here again. That's great motivation for me to accept the job. It also paid at the next grade higher than here, which impacted my retirement benefits."

A month after that conversation, just before 8 am at the beginning of my Surgical Committee meeting, Jim finally lost it.

"Do you realize how much money I've spent on your office furniture and computer, and how much I've spent in sending you to professional meetings?" "I'm going to release you from here on September second," he said.

"Jim, you're out of line. This is my meeting," I replied.

He railed on in front of other committee members, embarrassing me in front of my colleagues, and I immediately canceled the meeting.

His threat of a firm release date was especially troubling, since I did not yet have a finalized start date from Jackson, and a transferring federal employee cannot have a break in service without consequences. Those of you who grew up when I did know what the term "Indian Giver" means.

I now know the origin of that term.

Due to delays at the Jackson VA in processing my paperwork, I was not able to start there on September fifth. Government pay periods run in two week cycles, so I could not start there until September seventeenth. I had to go to Jim and ask him for a two-week extension on my employment in Browning.

"We already have another podiatrist available, but I guess I'll let you stay until then."

I doubted the validity of his statement regarding my replacement, as it took a year and a half to find me. This comment once again showed his lack of respect and knowledge of federal employment policies. It was also his way of humiliating me for leaving.

One of the most difficult situations I have ever encountered in my professional work occurred during my service as Chairman of the Surgical Committee. We had a group of contractors serving as nurse anesthetists (CRNA) who would work for a month at a time. One of these individuals came from Florida. He was a professional golfer and did anesthesia work mainly to supplement his earnings as a golfer. He was a fine anesthesia practitioner, and we worked together on a number of my surgical cases. One of our pharmacists was the daughter of another staff pharmacist. She was young and overzealous.

There appeared to be a discrepancy in accounting for controlled drugs used during surgery that was attributed to this particular anesthetist. All CRNAs were required to document usage and wasting of unused narcotics at the conclusion of every surgical case. Our particular accounting system for controlled drugs was different that what he was accustomed to at other hospitals, and he often neglected to properly record his drug wastage. This young pharmacist kept reporting this to me as Chairman of the Surgical Committee.

One day, she said to me, "I'm having trouble reconciling my records with his drug orders and the patient's chart." I replied,

"Have you double-checked all your paperwork and his?"

"I'll go back and check again just to be sure."

"You realize you may be placing this man in a difficult position if you're wrong."

She said, "I know."

I told her, "I'll speak to him myself about this."

I informally mentioned this to the CRNA who said, "This is a different system than I'm used to, but I'll work on it."

After several subsequent reports of alleged missing narcotics, the young pharmacist began to suspect that the CRNA might have been using them himself. I took up this issue with the Chief of Surgery. We agreed to meet with this nurse to discuss our concerns. The Chief said, "We're going to have to drug test him."

Both of us felt that this CRNA was not using drugs, but we felt compelled to follow through with our plan. One of the most awkward moments of my career occurred during this meeting in my office when I asked this nurse for a urine specimen. "I'll be happy to comply because I have nothing to hide," he said.

"I'm really sorry to have to put you through this." I said.

The Chief replied, "That goes for me too."

I personally took the sample to our lab, and spoke to the Chief of the lab. She said,

"I'll have to get permission from Jim to proceed."

Mr. Blackweasel denied payment for this test, and he was supported in his decision by the higher headquarters in Billings.

The test was never done.

The surgery chief and I felt terrible, and we apologized to this nurse. Needless to say, he never returned to Browning after that episode. We lost the services of a competent and decent CRNA. A while later, this same young pharmacist found the discrepancy as errors in her paperwork.

I subsequently focused the Surgical Committee's efforts at improving narcotics bookkeeping and prevention of this ever happening again. This pharmacist eventually left Browning for a position at Crow Agency near Billings.

* * *

Volunteerism was also alive and well in Browning. Each summer, a group of medical volunteers arrived from Chicago for a week. Included in this group was an orthopedist, who brought his entire staff and specialized equipment. A nurse practitioner at Browning coordinated the orthopedic care. He scheduled the routine knee and shoulder surgeries for that week, and followed them up after the volunteers leave. The orthopedist owned a ski chalet on Big Mountain, so he also came for a week in the winter during ski season.

These services were greatly appreciated by all, since orthopedic care was only directly available in Browning during those times. A group of family physicians and other specialists also from Chicago also volunteered the same week as the orthopedic group.

One day in July, I heard a knock at my door. As I opened the door, I saw a man I did not recognize. The man introduced himself.

"Hi, I'm Ron Wise, from Chicago. I teach dermatology at the Scholl Podiatry School."

He asked me, "Where did you go to school?"

"PCPM, or Temple as it's now called."

"Who did you have for dermatology?"

I replied, "Joe Witkowski."

"Joe and I go way back."

We hit it off immediately.

Ron and I were similar in age, and had much in common, including religion.

I had not heard a spoken Yiddish word in many years until he spoke a few to me. I must say it brought a warm, familiar feeling to me after living in a Christian and Native American world for so long. Dr. Wise presented two lunch time lectures to the staff at the hospital. These were the same lectures he gave to the podiatry students, and they were excellent.

We corresponded once after I arrived in Jackson, and I truly enjoyed my brief association with him. I missed his last lecture on a Friday, because I went to the emergency room as a patient with painful urinary retention.

The attending ER doctor sent in a nurse to catheterize me, much to my embarrassment and relief. The doctor's digital rectal exam revealed a much-enlarged prostate. Earlier in March, I had visited a urologist in Great Falls. He was procedure oriented, and wanted to do a prostate biopsy. I declined because I had no one to drive me from Great Falls after the procedure, and previous biopsies performed by my urologist in Ithaca were negative for cancer. The Great Falls urologist said during his digital rectal exam, "I don't feel any cancer."

I initially refused pain medication for the catheterization but after Linda heard my moans over the phone, they gave me pain meds. I left the ER catheterized and attached to a bag. A contract pharmacist from New Mexico stopped off at my quarters to check on me and asked, "Do you need anything from Costco?"

"Here's my grocery list. I really appreciate it."

Costco was in Kalispell, two hours away.

The next evening he dropped off some food I had ordered. That show of kindness and concern from him went a long way with me.

At about 6:15am on Sunday, I walked to the ER for removal of the catheter.

I believe the cause of my acute problem was triggered by dehydration during my hike to Grinnell Glacier in Glacier National Park the Sunday before.

Browning, MT was the worst place I had ever seen, let alone lived in. I had worked on several Indian reservations in New Mexico, and had casually observed the poverty and desperate conditions there while driving to and from the clinics for a day a month. I can recall dogs running loose on these reservations. Upon entering town from the east, one passes the Town Pump, a Montana franchise that sold gas, beer, and other sundries. The Browning store sold the most Bud Light of any store in the state.

Proceeding west on Highway Two, one passes closed businesses and other buildings in disrepair. Turning right on Piegan Street to go to the hospital, Icks bar was on the left. At any given time of day or night, the drunks stood outside this establishment waiting for who knows what.

Browning had one grocery store, the I.G.A., no retail pharmacy, no movie theater, no dry cleaners, no McDonalds, a Subway, Taco Johns, two other sit down restaurants, a Chinese and Mexican restaurant, two gift shops, and two gas stations with only one working air hose (sometimes). There was a pawn shop, a dollar store, the Native American Bank, U.S. Post Office, a Catholic church, and the public schools. There were two hardware stores (not Lowes or Home Depot). Browning Lumber and Hardware was where the local maintenance department hung out when not on coffee breaks.

Panhandling by natives outside the IGA or Post Office was a common unpleasant event. I eventually learned to ignore it. Browning also boasted a new thirteen-million-dollar casino that was nearly empty most of the time. Within three months of its opening, the casino laid off one hundred sixty employees.

The Tribal mentality was, "If you build it, they will come".

Of course, Mr. and Mrs. Middle America from Iowa who planned their annual summer family vacation to visit Glacier National Park were not going to drop a quarter into a slot machine at the casino, let alone play other games of chance with their hard-earned vacation money. The thirteen million dollars would have been better spent on a teen recreation center or SPCA facility. No one ever asked my opinion, but I could have told him or her so.

Hard core gamblers, including other Blackfeet traveled to bigger Indian casinos in Idaho or to Las Vegas.

Linda, who always has a creative spin to her thinking, once asked me,

"Evan, do you think they used the casino to launder drug money?"

"I really don't know."

Perhaps the best of Browning aside from its geography was the Museum of the Plains Indians, currently financed by the U.S. government but became tribal. A decent art gallery was across the street. I was told that thirty years ago, Browning was a nice place, with many more prosperous white-owned businesses that catered to residents and summer tourists (there are no winter tourists). The town had been on a continued downhill slide.

Browning Lumber was the one remaining white owned business, as the corrupt Tribal Council has discouraged non-native owned businesses over the years. The constant winds in Browning are an untapped energy resource.

One of my patients was the son of an unsuccessful candidate who ran for a position on the Tribal Council. His dad's platform was based on attracting a large energy company to build wind turbines on the reservation. He actually had a firm multimillion dollar commitment from that company, but he lost the election.

My patient said, "The Tribal Council is corrupt. They want to keep the rest of the tribe poor so they can line their own pockets."

That worthy project would have brought much needed wealth and prosperity to the Blackfeet Nation, not to mention a great source of clean energy.

All of this squalor is situated among one of the most spectacular panoramas of the mountains of Glacier National Park to the west and the Great Plains to the east. Browning is the gateway to the east entrance to Glacier National Park, and to the approach to St. Mary and Many Glacier area of the Park to the north towards the Canadian border.

The weather in Browning was usually better than the weather in the mountains or on the west side (Whitefish, Kalispell). Browning was just twelve miles east of the Front Range of the Rockies. Most of the moisture from the Pacific Northwest drops on the west side of the high mountains before reaching Browning, hence, it is sunnier.

Browning was also one of the windiest places in the US. It is common to have sustained wind speeds of sixty to eighty mph, with gusts to over one-hundred-twenty mph. Of course, winds of this magnitude can and do cause structural damage. I can recall observing my SUV rock back and forth in my driveway during one of those wind storms. Quarters number twelve was a two-story building built in 1988. It was poorly built then, and even more poorly maintained. One night, wind gusts exceeded one-hundred-twenty mph, and my building creaked and groaned. I went to the basement for shelter. That storm blew siding off several other similar houses to mine. Hurricane ratings begin as Category 1 with sustained wind speeds of 75 mph.

On another rainy night, I awoke to a dripping sound in the spare bedroom, where I had my desk and computer. I noticed water on the computer, and discovered a leak in my ceiling. I thought, "One of the basic requirements of housing is to have a secure roof over your head. Is that asking too much?"

I quickly moved my valuables out of harm's way, and placed an empty bucket under the leaky spot. After reporting the damage the next day, my maintenance man "fixed" the leak in the roof with DUCT TAPE! Needless to say, it leaked again during the next rain.

The Duct Tape Company had an online contest for people to submit stories of how they used their product. I did not win, but I thought my entry was descriptive but embellished a little in hopes of winning. Here was my entry:

> Browning, Montana is situated along the Front Range of the northern Rocky Mountains twelve miles from the east entrance to Glacier National Park. It is one of the windiest places in the US. It is not unusual to get a 'stiff breeze' of eighty to one-hundred-twenty mph. In some parts of the US winds of this magnitude are called hurricanes. A few years ago, the wind blew the Amtrak train off the track in East Glacier Park, Montana. A fence was built on the downwind side of the railroad bridge

> over Midvale Creek to prevent future trains from ending up in the water. I do not know if they used duct tape to build this fence, but it is still standing.
>
> I developed a leak in my roof. The Indian Health Service is an underfunded federal agency, so duct tape is a popular and inexpensive was to fix things around the reservation. Unable to afford a new roof or the correct repair required, the Blackfeet maintenance man used his trusty roll of duct tape to fix the leak. Hats (not roofs) off to duct tape.

The part about the train blowing off the tracks is true.

Browning has enormous potential as a gateway town to the Park if the Tribal Council ever decided to allow healthy development.

The Blackfeet Reservation is over two thousand three hundred square miles in size; larger than the state of Delaware. The woefully understaffed Bureau of Indian Affairs (BIA) carried out Law enforcement. The local BIA officers were related to most on the reservation, making impartial law enforcement impossible. The local Glacier County Sheriff and the Montana State Patrol were only permitted on state and US highways that pass through the reservation. Even the FBI only had limited jurisdiction, and only with capital murder cases. In Browning, one could literally get away with murder and drug dealing was rampant.

Montana is the fourth largest state by area, but had less than a million residents. Until the late 1990's, there was no maximum speed limit. The federal government threatened to cut the state's revenues unless they agreed to institute a speed limit. The open container law was just recently passed. Until then, it was legal to have an open container of alcohol in your vehicle while driving.

Montana ranked fourth in the nation behind the District of Columbia, Rhode Island, and Massachusetts with the highest rates of driving under the influence of illicit drugs. (Office of Applied Studies . (2007). Changes in Prevalence Rates of Drug Use between 2002-2003 and 2004-2005 among states. Rockville, MD: Substance Abuse and Mental Health Services Administration).

The Blackfeet reservation had an open range policy for livestock. Horses and cattle were allowed to roam freely across roadways. If you hit one with your vehicle, you were responsible for all financial losses to the owner, if you survived the crash. The chances of survival after striking a twelve-hundred-pound horse at seventy-five mph are not good, and one of our staff lost her husband in just such an encounter. Elk, deer, moose, and bears are commonly encountered crossing roadways. I had a few close calls myself with both wild and domestic animals.

During our first trip to Kalispell after Linda arrived in May, Linda screamed,

"Watch out for the deer!"

"Yes, dear."

I slalomed our Mountaineer SUV through a heard of seven deer that were crossing Route 2 just east of West Glacier. I attribute my successful maneuvering to my well- honed skiing skills perfected on the slopes of Big Mountain the previous winter. Alcohol and drug abuse was widespread in Montana. When you combine these factors with severe weather and mountainous terrain you have the most dangerous driving conditions I have ever encountered. Highway 2 in Montana contributed to this state's having had the highest fatality rate in the country (National Highway Transportation and Safety Administration, 2010).

I was driving back to Browning one Sunday evening after a weekend of skiing at Big Mountain. The weather was fine as I approached West Glacier. Snow flurries soon turned into an all-out blizzard as my SUV climbed toward Marias Pass and the Continental Divide. I was about one-quarter-of-a-mile behind another car, traveling at a sensible speed for these conditions and well below the posted speed limit as I approached a curve. The road curved left, but my Mountaineer stayed straight and I bounced off a guard rail. Even my skiing ability could not have saved me from that accident. I was actually inside Glacier National Park near Bear Creek where there was no cell phone coverage and little traffic. My vehicle was still drivable and I made it to Browning safely. I had the SUV repaired in Great Falls while I was in Texas visiting Linda.

I never told her about the accident.

My insurance company claimed the accident was my fault because I lost control of my vehicle and wanted to raise my rates. I am a veteran snow and ice driver from Upstate New York. During a phone call with the insurance company, I said, "Even Bobby Unser himself could not have avoided that accident."

After speaking to a senior executive with the company, he said, "Dr. Meltzer, you've been a loyal customer of our company for many years. Because of that, we will not raise your rates over this accident.

Gary Barker, a U S Public Health Service Captain was assigned to be Chief of Pharmacy in Browning. Harold welcomed his arrival, and was relieved at stepping down from the hot seat as acting chief. Gary moved from an Indian Health Service facility in Ketchikan, Alaska. While driving from Kalispell to Browning in his brand-new Ford F-250 truck, he hit an icy patch of road and struck the guard rails on the opposite side of the road near an outhouse next to recreational access to the Middle Fork of the Flathead River on Highway Two. The guard rails stayed damaged through the following summer. The state of Montana charged Gary's insurance company twelve thousand dollars to eventually repair the guard rails.

Even Harold, the Montana native and veteran Highway Two driver struck the guard rail with his ten-year-old Honda Civic on his way home one Friday night, not far from my accident site. Fortunately, none of us were injured and we shared a common bond as a result. When I lived in New Mexico, I called it the Wild West. I think of Montana as the Wild, Wild West.

* * *

Wildfires are another fact of life in the West. When I was a boy, they were called forest fires. Smokey the Bear would say in his deep animated voice during the black-and-white TV commercials of the 1950s, "Only You Can Prevent Forest Fires".

I learned much later that Smokey was a real black bear that was found alive but badly burned after a forest fire in Lincoln County, New Mexico (also where Billy the Kid was jailed).

Every spring, all primary care providers at the hospital performed firefighting physical exams. Seasonal firefighting was one of the main sources of income to the Blackfeet and both men and women participate. Blackfeet crews can be sent anywhere in the US to fight wildfires if they are needed. A significant number of Blackfeet also assisted in the Hurricane Katrina cleanup.

In July, Linda and I were traveling back to Browning from a podiatry meeting at the Big Sky Resort near Bozeman. We were about thirty miles south of Browning when we noticed a large plume of smoke on the horizon. Linda said, "Maybe Browning is on fire".

We both laughed at that possibility, as that would be one dramatic way to obliterate the ramshackle buildings in town. As I looked more closely, I said, "It looks like the smoke is coming from the St. Mary area."

It turns out I was correct.

Upon our arrival at home, we could see plumes of smoke coming from just below Divide Mountain on the south shore of St. Mary Lake. That night, we could see flames erupting as trees exploded thirty miles away. The Red Eagle Fire eventually consumed over thirty-three thousand acres-about half in Glacier National Park and the other half on the reservation. The Forest Service and National Park Service had adopted new firefighting concepts after the devastating 1988 Yellowstone fire. Since the fire in the Park was not a threat to any structures, it was allowed to burn out. The eastern half across the highway burned some valuable timber on the reservation.

Fire suppression was employed to save structures in the town of St. Mary, and a tent fire camp was established just outside of town. Roads were closed to St. Mary for a time. Weeks later, just before we left for Texas, we drove through the area. The pavement on Route Forty-Nine was scorched black where the fire jumped the road to the reservation on the east side of the road. The devastation was complete. The cause of the Red Eagle Fire was never determined. The Blackfeet Tribe harvested about one-million dollars in timber from standing burned trees the following summer.

The following summer, the Skyland Fire burned about thirty-five-thousand acres, consuming the trees surrounding our popular ski road/trail. That fire was determined to be caused by lightning. Smokey was wrong on that one-we could not have prevented it. Harold, another pharmacist and I drove up to and over Marias Pass to observe the fire and associated activity. There were still small brush fires next to the highway that were left to burn. Route Two was closed to traffic periodically as the fire changed course. This is the main highway west from Browning to Kalispell.

The alternate route was through St. Mary and over the Going-To-The-Sun Road in the Park- a sixty-mile detour. One Saturday morning, Route Two was open, and I drove my Mountaineer to Kalispell to sell it to a dealer. The contract pharmacist from New Mexico agreed to meet me at the dealership, and we would drive back to Browning together. After our usual Costco run and socializing at Harold and Pam's house, we left there about 10pm. We drove past West Glacier on Route Two, and about five miles from Marias Pass we were turned around by a local officer. It was about 11:30 by then, and we were both tired. "Do you feel you can drive to Browning tonight?" I asked him.

"I'm tired, but I don't want to pay for a room in West Glacier."

The only way back was to reverse our course back to West Glacier and over the Going-To-The-Sun Road. The West entrance to the Park was manned twenty four/seven during the high season, so they could collect the entrance fee.

Charging a fee did not seem fair for those who were actually using the Road for commuting and not sightseeing. Fortunately, I had my Glacier Park pass for the season. It was an otherwise beautiful night with a full moon. My driver had actually never been over the Road before. We stopped briefly at Logan Pass to take in the dramatic sight of the surrounding moonlit mountains.

"This is really beautiful," he said.

Cyclists like to ride the Road at night during a full moon, and we found ourselves pulling over his Jeep towards the steep drop-offs to allow the bicycles to pass safely. It was an eerie sight to see a line of bright single headlamps descend the Road at midnight. I concluded this was not a safe thing to do and decided that adventure would not make my "Bucket List." I got dropped off about 2am at my quarters.

I am a lifetime member of the Michigan State University Alumni Association. I planned to meet with a University official in Kalispell who was vacationing there. We were planning to meet for dinner. The Skyland Fire caused the closure of Route Two that day, and I did not want to drive the one hundred twenty extra miles round trip of detour over the Going-To-The-Sun Road just for dinner.

I do not recommend driving the Road at night after a few drinks.

I was disappointed to have to miss that event.

The Blackfeet Community Hospital provides free inpatient and outpatient medical care and prescription and non-prescription drugs to all enrolled Native residents. It was the second busiest Emergency Department in the State, with helicopter and fixed wing air ambulance service available twenty-four/seven at five to seven thousand dollars per trip. Arguably, the most scenic helicopter ride in the US is from Browning to Kalispell- directly over Glacier National Park. I always wanted a ride, but not as a patient. The hospital is staffed by a variety of employees. My job description did not list me as officially on call, but I lived within a short walk from the ER. The ER docs were my friends and neighbors, and they would call me if they needed my services anytime they knew I was around. Again, as a Title Five employee, I could count the time I spent outside my normal duty hours as overtime pay or as compensatory time for leave.

One Easter morning, I had just finished showering. There was a knock on my door.

A hospital ambulance was in my driveway. The driver said, "Dr. Ender wants you to come to the ER immediately."

"He could have just called; I don't need a ride in an ambulance."

I called Dr. Ender to ask about the patient, and he told me I might need to take him to the operating room. I said, "I'll be right over. Please notify the OR staff they might need to come in."

I quickly dressed and walked, not rode to the ER. After examining the patient, I determined he did not require surgery.

The US Public Health Service has assigned some uniformed professionals, including physicians, optometrists, dentists, pharmacists, lab technicians and others to work at the Indian Health Service. Other non-native professionals like me are government employees of the Indian Health Service, under the Department of Health and Human Services. There were also a large number of contract employees mostly in the nursing area. These people have to renegotiate their contracts on a regular basis which was a major inconvenience to them.

Karen Green was one of those employees, and I had to write her several letters of recommendation each time her contract expired. She had worked there for over twenty years under this system.

The infrastructure and staff was in place to deliver excellent medical and dental care to any eligible resident (called "bens" for beneficiaries). Unfortunately, the Blackfeet were not a healthy group, and many did not avail themselves of the excellent resource.

Diabetes was rampant among Native Americans, and my salary was subsidized through a grant from the Southern Peigan Diabetes Project. The hospital also had a chronic pain clinic that was run by a now-retired physician and his job was taken over by a nurse practitioner. After the doctor retired, the nurse (Blackfeet wife of the Glacier County Sheriff) ran the clinic herself, without physician oversight. This contributed to the fueling of an illegal drug trade of prescription narcotics. The pharmacists unofficially called Friday "narc day", as the addicts sought to get their supply for self use and for sale over the weekend. It was commonplace to see drug transactions take place between parked cars in Browning on Friday evenings. The street value of a Percocet tablet was reported to be twenty dollars.

The pharmacists in general and Harold in particular were strongly against this unsupervised nurse practitioner and her pain clinic.

I routinely prescribed Percocet to my post-operative patients, and been doing so for the past thirty years. One of my patients who lived in Babb, Montana about forty miles from Browning near the Canadian border told me an incredible story on her first post-operative visit. She said a man came from Browning to ask her for her pain medication. I asked her, "Who was this man?"

"He was a cousin, but I didn't give him any of my pills because I didn't know how many I might need," she replied.

After thirty years of podiatric surgical practice, this was a first for me.

We lived in a loop area near the Emergency Department with other families and hospital employees. The assistant hospital CEO lived with his family and six children in a three-bedroom house just like ours. Traffic would come and go in front of their house day and night. Linda openly saw drug deals go down between one of this man's sons and customers. Grandpa would sit in a lawn chair smoking a cigarette with a shotgun across his lap and keeping watch. As long as he stayed on the reservation, drug enforcement could not touch him. This and other reservations are considered sovereign nations. Linda felt unsafe in the neighborhood, and she suggested," Why don't you drop a hint to Tim that the Meltzer's are armed citizens?"

I asked, "How should I do that?"

"Why don't you ask him where we can find a good place to shoot our guns."?

I approached Tim the next day with that question. "Tim, Linda and I have pistols, and we're wondering where we can go around here to practice."

"I think there's a range over in Cut Bank."

He was an educated man, and I'm sure my underlying reason for asking that question was not lost on him. We never had any trouble from his family.

Tim's next-door neighbor was an ER nurse, who had over fifty guns locked in a safe at his quarters. He actually warned one of Tim's kids who was waving a gun around outside towards his house.

"If you ever point a gun at my house again, I'll shoot back."

He never had any more trouble after that either.

* * *

Certain holiday celebrations were quite interesting in Browning. For my first Halloween, Linda left me with what she thought was the usual amount of candy I would need for the Trick or Treaters we had been used to. Within about fifteen minutes, all my candy was gone. At least two hundred sugar-addicted, poor children pounded on my door until nine pm begging for candy for themselves, their siblings, friends, and their baby brothers and sisters in the car. Parents lined their cars up at the entrance to our circle of houses and were gridlocked along the entire road.

The following year, I was determined not to create any more business for our overworked dentists, and Linda sent me a large box of plastic toys I could give away instead of candy. Fortunately, I had enough of those treasures to last the evening.

July fourth celebrations usually began about two weeks before, with nightly fireworks going off at all hours. As the actual date approached, the bombardment escalated. I have not experienced combat first hand, but believe that Browning came close to mimicking a town under siege. I called the local BIA (Bureau of Indian Affairs) office on several occasions to complain about the noise, but got little response. As I previously mentioned, most of the Officers were related to the perpetrators. Finally, one night before I had three surgical cases to perform, I called and complained,

"How would you like to be the patient of a sleep-deprived surgeon?"

That tactic was successful.

The real irony was that these Indians were celebrating a holiday that represented the independence of the country that mistreated them for so many years. The cost of fireworks was also considerable. One lady told me she had money withheld from her paycheck to pay for fireworks. Most Blackfeet did not have that money to burn.

One day I was treating a woman in my clinic. She told me, "Some members of the Tribal Council say you are racist."

I replied, "That's crap. I'm the minority here."

"Do you really think I would live and work in this town if I really felt that way?"

She absorbed my comments, and said, "I guess not."

The Blackfeet were equal opportunity racists, even among themselves. Tribal members who spent considerable time living off the reservation in metropolitan areas such as Seattle, Portland, or even in Missoula or Great Falls were referred to as "Apples"; "Red on the outside and white on the inside." The Blackfeet also had a term for homosexuals; they refer to them as "Two-Spirited."

The reality was that many Blackfeet hated the white folks, but begrudgingly accepted them because there are not enough educated Indians to fill all the highly skilled positions at the hospital. As a result, as dangerous as Browning can be at night, hospital employees were rarely bothered except by the panhandlers at the IGA. One day I was out for a walk after work. I was walking in one of the other housing areas when a crazed young Indian man began yelling at me, "Hey you! You there!"

We were walking in the same general direction, and I realized he would soon intersect with my path. There was no one else in sight. Fortunately, I was headed in the direction of the hospital, and I bolted for the Emergency Room.

He did not follow me. He was clearly high on some drug, probably methamphetamine.

During the last six months of my tenure in Browning, there were a series of revealing articles in the Great Falls Tribune regarding the illicit trade of controlled substances in Browning. This predictably got the attention of the Drug Enforcement Administration, which has oversight of the hospital's DEA number. The week I left, two physicians, the hospital CEO and the Chief of Pharmacy were ordered to a meeting in Billings with officials from the DEA's Denver office to discuss remediation policies relating to excessive narcotics use on the reservation. According to the DEA, Browning's consumption of controlled substances was seven times the normal amount for a community of that size (about nine thousand). The DEA is a branch of the Department of Justice and has all the enforcement powers it requires to rescind licenses and prescribing abilities of institutions and providers. They also have the power of arrest. I do not know the outcome of those meetings, but am relieved that my association with this hospital no longer threatened my license or my ability to prescribe controlled medication.

* * *

There was no local mail delivery in Browning, Montana. Every resident was issued a free Post Office box. Unlike most Post Offices around the country, the Browning office locked its doors promptly at 5:30pm to limit access to the drunks and homeless attempting to stay warm. I usually drove to the Post Office during my lunch hour, since I worked until 5:30pm. When Linda was living with me in Browning, she would make the mail run.

One day, she told me, "An Indian man exposed himself to me at the Post Office."

"Really."

"I was opening our mailbox and as I turned around, he dropped his pants right in front of me." We laughed.

"Was there much to see?

I was shocked, but not surprised. Linda was disgusted.

I always picked up the mail after that incident.

I cannot recall how or when I met Harold. He was acting chief of the pharmacy but was also a third generation Montana wheat farmer. He worked four ten-hour days in the hospital pharmacy Tuesday-Friday, living in government quarters adjacent to the hospital. On Friday night-Monday, he went home to his wife, Pam and his farm near Kalispell in the beautiful and fertile Flathead Valley. We quickly became close friends.

Harold was born in October of 1946 in Kalispell, a fellow baby boomer. He lived with Pam in a home less than a mile from his ninety-five-year-old mother and the land he grew up on and also geographically close to his sisters. Harold was in the farming business with his younger brother Phil until Phil's death. His other younger brother was a disabled pharmacist.

Throughout my travels in the US, I have always been fascinated with others born in 1946. Regardless of our upbringing and background, we all shared the same American cultural experience growing up as fellow baby boomers. These common experiences are so well described in the various works of one of my favorite authors, fellow baby boomer and humorist Dave Barry of Miami.

In spite of our ethnic differences, a Jewish kid from Rochester shares this common ground with a Montana descendant of a German immigrant like Harold to a Hispanic from New Mexico, a Blackfeet Indian from Montana or an African-American from Mississippi. Because I was in the medical field, I was constantly comparing myself with my contemporaries. "Do I look older or younger? Am I as healthy or less well?"

I considered them all my spiritual classmates; high school class of 1964; college class of 1968 for those fortunate enough to have gone to college. Harold was a 1968 graduate of the University of Montana.

Harold and I shared many other things in common. He was an Army veteran like me, and was working towards the same government retirement goal as I am. He was a fellow professional, and worked full-time as a pharmacist at the Blackfeet hospital. His other full-time job was wheat farmer.

Harold grew up in the shadow of Big Mountain in Whitefish, so he had his fill of downhill skiing as a younger man. He gave up that sport for cross country skiing, a sport I had not done for many years. Downhill skiing is still my passion, but Harold's enthusiasm for cross country got me back into that healthy sport again. I made Harold a sign for his desk at work, declaring him "Director of Nordic Skiing at Blackfeet Community Hospital".

He was the creator and founder of the "Young and the Restless" ski club of Browning. Harold and I were the first of the Restless group. Every month throughout the year, groups of senior pharmacy students mainly from Samford University in Birmingham, Alabama would spend one-month clinical externships at the hospital. Many had never even seen snow before, let alone had ever skied.

Harold was always buying used ski equipment in Kalispell or Whitefish, and brought it with him to Browning. He had enough variety and sizes crammed into his quarters to fit any male or female student who wanted to ski. These young and enthusiastic students took to cross country skiing easily, although some of the Southern Belles did not do well with the cold weather. Harold had boundless energy, and was always trying to arrange ski trips after work.

He would often be heard saying on a cold winter night, "Let's mount an expedition for tonight."

Unfortunately, his ten-hour days never ended before 7pm, and by the time dinner was scarfed down and we drove to our destination, it might be around 9pm or later before we would be sliding along with our headlamps lighting the way.

Cross country skiing is one of the top conditioning sports one can participate in. Upper and lower body strength and balance are developed, along with aerobic cardiovascular fitness. It can even be fun. Although I much preferred downhill skiing and cross-country skiing during daylight, most of my cross-country skiing was done at night with Harold and crew.

We had several places to go skiing depending on the snow conditions. Global warming has affected Montana. The Browning locals reported that winters were much more severe years ago, with snow levels in previous winters measured in feet in Browning itself.

The two winters I spent in Browning, snow accumulation in town was minimal, so we would have to travel to higher elevations to find snow for skiing. One popular place was Marias Pass, the Continental Divide at about five-thousand-three hundred feet above sea level. This was twenty miles west of Browning. The Autumn Creek trail was across the railroad tracks, and went into the Park. Grizzly bear sightings were common on this trail. Another popular area was Isaac Walton Inn at Essex, forty miles west of Browning.

They had miles of lighted and groomed cross country ski trails located behind the Inn. If we arrived before 8pm, we could get a good dinner at the Inn before skiing. We would often finish skiing at 10:30-11pm, share a bottle of wine in the parking lot, and then drive back to Browning.

Needless to say, sleep would be sacrificed for fun, exercise and camaraderie.

We also skied on the road to Two Medicine Lake just outside of East Glacier. There was a short, steep road from that one going down to the lake. Once we hit the lake, we could ski for miles on the snow and ice covered lake with breathtaking moonlit views of the surrounding mountains.

One February night, we heard the distant sounds of the air ambulance helicopter flying from Kalispell to Browning to pick up a sick or injured patient. I came to call this service, "Harry's Helicopters," after Harry Ender, MD. Harry worked twelve hour shifts in the emergency room on weekends and had a small apartment adjacent to the hospital. Like Harold, he went home to his wife and family in Kalispell during the week.

Another favorite place to ski was on the golf course and surrounding grounds of the Glacier Park Lodge in East Glacier. This was the closest place to Browning for skiing, and minimized our drive time. I was often the driver, as my capable four-wheel drive Mercury Mountaineer was large enough to carry four skiers and all our gear. I dubbed it "Meltzer's Skiwagen."

On one night there, the snow was so deep we skied across the top of the picnic tables, enjoying the moment. One evening the next summer while lounging on the deck of the Lodge admiring the panoramic view of the mountains, Harold struck up a conversation with one of the guests.

"Where are you from?"

"I'm from South Carolina."

"Are you enjoying your visit to the Park?"

"You bet, we went hiking today."

"See those picnic tables over there? My friend and I skied across them last winter."

The young man's eyes widened at his remark. "That's cool; we don't see much snow back home"

I really felt like a local that night.

The Skyland Trail just over Marias Pass was another popular ski trail. This road leads to a creek and into the Bob Marshall Wilderness Area. This trail was all uphill for the entire way we would ski it-about two or three miles. The trip back down hill was fun especially with deep powder snow. I fell on my ski pole and broke it on my first outing there. One night Harold and I were skiing at this spot. Harold was way ahead of me as usual. He has long legs and good ski technique, and he was the hare while I was the tortoise. As I was chugging my way uphill, I heard a crash in the surrounding forest. I did not detect any movement, nor did I see any animal tracks, but it unnerved me. I yelled,

"Harold, turn around, I'm freaked out".

It was on a rare Saturday during the day that Harold and I skied the Bear Creek drainage area, a bit further west of the Skyland Trail. Harold had to work that weekend at the pharmacy. In his usual form, Harold sped ahead of me. I reached a fork in the trail and followed where I thought he had gone. We lost each other for about an hour in broad daylight. After that adventure, I bought a pair of walkie-talkies that I took on every subsequent ski trip.

As mentioned, the Autumn Creek Trail was across the railroad tracks from the summit of Marias Pass. This track was the major rail route from Chicago to Portland and Seattle, with as many as thirty-five trains per day passing through, including the daily Amtrak. The rail cars would be full of western grain headed for Minneapolis.

On one dark night, the Young and Restless crew crossed over the tracks to ski on the Trail. I found the icy trail conditions especially treacherous, I said to Harold, "It's too icy for me, I'm afraid I might break something."

"We'll meet you back at your rig. Be careful crossing the tracks."

We had another contract pharmacist with us from Dallas, and he wasn't too pleased with the ski conditions either. He said, "Evan, I'm coming with you."

As we skied toward the tracks, an eastbound train slowed and stopped, blocking our way to my vehicle. We took off our skis and hesitated for a few minutes.

I decided to take a chance hoping the train would not move.

I climbed between two rail cars-first by laying my skis onto the coupling between the cars and then quickly climbing over to the other side and grabbing my skis. The other guy freaked out. "Evan, I can't do this," he said.

"Yes you can, just do it quickly in case the train starts to move."

He stood on the other side of the train for a few minutes, frozen in fear.

"Look, you have to climb over now. Hand me your skis."

I climbed back onto the coupling and quickly grabbed his skis. I climbed down even more quickly. We had no way of knowing when or if the train would suddenly move.

Finally, he decided he'd better act.

I assisted him from my side. Fortunately, the train remained parked.

It was not our time.

The Great Northern Railway was largely responsible for opening up Glacier National Park to tourists. To promote business, the Great Northern built most of the great lodges in the Park, including East Glacier and Many Glacier Lodges. Glacier became an official National Park in 1910, but tourists had been arriving there for years prior to its official designation.

The Amtrak train from Chicago to Portland was called the Empire Builder. In summer, the train stops at the town of East Glacier. One can actually walk from the train station to Glacier Park Lodge. From fall until early May, the train also stops in Browning. In summer, the train was full of tourists from the east headed for the Park and points west.

In May, I was on one of my trips to visit Linda in Texas. For twelve dollars, I took the Empire Builder from Browning to Whitefish. My hotel transportation in Whitefish was waiting for me at the train station, and also took me to the Glacier airport in Kalispell early the next morning. The two-hour train ride goes right through the Park, stopping at the Isaac Walton Inn in Essex and at West Glacier before arriving at Whitefish.

Riding in the glass domed railcars was a great experience. It was difficult to appreciate the scenery along Highway Two while driving along the same route.

One notable adventure occurred just prior to my getting Linda from Texas. Carl was another pharmacist at the hospital. His daughter Jeannette was also the young pharmacist who stirred up the trouble with the contract nurse anesthetist. Carl lived in Cut Bank, and owned his own airplane. He also owned his own hangar at the Cut Bank airport where he kept it. Cut Bank was a decaying town just east of the Blackfeet reservation that boomed during the 1980s from oil revenues. I can remember from years past hearing weather reports that Cut Bank, Montana was the coldest spot in the U.S. on that particular winter day.

One evening Harold invited me to a barbeque and plane ride at Carl's hangar. Harold and Phil were in the farming business together as Clarke Brothers. Phil was sick for years with heart disease, and Harold was determined to live a healthier lifestyle. This was one reason he was so passionate about cross country skiing. Harold was unusually quiet during the drive to Cut Bank. Finally, he said,

"My brother died today".

"Harold, I'm very sorry."

With the usual entourage of pharmacy students, we met Carl at the airport. The grill faire was elk steaks from last fall's hunt from

Carl's freezer. Before sunset, Carl took turns taking the students and us on short rides in his Cessna with breathtaking views of the Front Range. We flew over a Hutterite colony and Carl did a few touch-and-go landings. After we helped him secure the plane in the hangar, we feasted on the steaks, enjoying beer and Crown Royal. Harold talked about Carl's flying us into the Great Bear Wilderness on the west side of the mountains for a steak roast and camp out.

It was a memorable evening.

Carl was a cautious pilot with great respect for mountain weather. We never made that Great Bear trip happen.

First winter without Linda

Linda suffers from several health problems that make her unable to tolerate extreme cold. We were also attempting to sell our Texas home so we could look for a house or building lot in Montana. For those reasons, Linda had to stay in Texas where the climate is warmer, and to attend to the showing of the house. We were not happy about being geographically separated, but that was our reality.

My first weekend alone in Montana felt odd. I was totally free of any family responsibilities, dog-walking, and home maintenance chores. All that remained was work, recreation and self amusement. Someone had to do it! I drove up to Two Medicine Lake on Saturday prepared to go hiking. Hiking alone in Glacier or Yellowstone Parks is not recommended, due to the prevalence of grizzly bears. I grew up as a Boy Scout hiking in the Adirondack Mountains of northern New York State. We learned to hike quietly so we could observe wildlife along the way.

The Adirondacks does have its share of black bears, but they are shy creatures seldom seen along hiking trails. Hiking while making as much noise as possible was initially counter-intuitive for me. Grizzly bears are also normally shy, but can be unpredictable. A family doctor at the hospital who had been there for over twenty years told me stories of several patients he had treated over the years after being mauled by a grizzly. I remained cautious and respectful of Ursus Horribilus.

As I was getting ready to hike the trail around Two Medicine Lake in Glacier Park, a noisy family started down the same trail. I decided to shadow them and let them be the noise makers I needed. Since they had small children, I quickly overtook them and was soon on my own. I occasionally shouted out,

"Hey bear!"

I also sung a few old songs as loud as I could. As I climbed higher up the trail, I realized I was totally alone. While I relished the solitude, I also felt uneasy by myself.

It was common for hikers to carry jingle bells on their packs as noise makers. The locals joke and call them "dinner bells", for all the good they do. Bells always worked for me, as I never had a close encounter with a bear.

As of this writing, no one other than park rangers were permitted to carry firearms in a national park. The only personal defense one was allowed to carry is bear spray. This is a large can of pepper spray (capsaisin) that can discourage a bear if you are within range.

I had decided years ago to be an armed citizen, and would rather deal with the legal system and live than be dead. In direct violation of Park rules, I always carried my loaded Glock forty-caliber pistol deep in my pack, but accessible if needed. Fortunately, I never needed to use the pistol or bear spray.

As autumn came to a close, I was anxiously awaiting the opening of Big Mountain Ski Resort. I had not been downhill skiing for two and a half years, and planned to purchase all new equipment that season. I purchased new ski boots and skis at a ski shop in Whitefish in late fall. Equipment changes rapidly in this sport, and I wanted to begin the season with all new gear. Although my equipment was ready and new, my fifty-nine- year-old body was out of shape for skiing. I showed up on opening day at Big Mountain in early December with my new gear and old body.

One of the nicknames of Big Mountain was "Fog Mountain." The mountains of western Montana frequently get moist air from the Pacific, creating many days of clouds and fog on the western slopes. Browning is on the eastern Front Range, and most of the moisture is dropped on the western slopes by the time the air mass reaches the Front Range. Visibility on Big Mountain was often measured in "chair" units, that is, how many lift chairs you can see ahead of you on the chair lift. On opening day, visibility was only one or two chairs. The rest were lost in the fog. So here I was, on a new mountain, with bad visibility, untested equipment, and a de-conditioned body. Fortunately, I am an experienced skier with a long history of skiing at many resorts in both the east and west under all weather conditions.

I took the chair lift to the summit, and looked for a blue trail. Ski trails are graded with green circles (easiest), blue squares (intermediate), black diamonds (advanced), double black diamonds (expert), and in the case of Jackson Hole in 1986, yellow triangles (suicidal). There are no standards comparing slopes of one resort with another. What slopes are green at one mountain might be equivalent to blue at another, etc.

I survived the first blue trail, and soon realized my boots were killing my big toes, my legs were woefully out of shape, and my new skis would take some getting used to. After a few painful runs, I decided to call it a day and return to the ski shop for some boot adjustments. It was so foggy, I asked a fellow skier,

"Can you help me find the way down to the main lodge?"

Trail maps were useless in the thick pea soup fog of that day, and I followed him down the trail.

After my first day, I went back to the shop in Whitefish for a boot adjustment. I skied in those ill-fitting boots for the remainder of the season, causing loss of both big toenails. Multiple attempts by the boot fitter at the shop could not provide the proper fit I needed. I finally traded in these new boots for a different brand that fit me well, and made my second ski season much more comfortable.

* * *

Thanksgiving was spent away from Linda. This was our first ever Thanksgiving apart. She volunteered to serve the festive meal at a soup kitchen in Texas while I was invited to dinner at the Wagner home in the government quarters complex. Steve Wagner, MD lived with his wife, Anna and two kids at the time. Anna was pregnant with their third. Steve was director of the Emergency Department, and also a board-certified pediatrician.

The Wagners' came to Browning directly out of Steve's residency to work for a few years in the Indian Health Service for debt relief. Every year of work in the Indian Health Service reduced his student debt by a certain amount. The Wagners' had always planned to do medical missionary work in Africa, and were in the process of arranging for that part of their lives when I left Browning. They were gracious and friendly hosts, always inviting wayward souls like myself for holiday dinners. They were also best friends with our mutual neighbors, the Hind family.

Justine and Alan were neighbors who moved to Browning from Ann Arbor, Michigan. Justine was a Physician Assistant who had been recruited by Jonie Hind. Alan had recently retired after a thirty-year career at General Motors, and had just enrolled in nursing school in Michigan. The four of us became good friends.

Alan and Linda got to know each other during the day while Justine and I worked at the hospital. Justine was put in charge of administering cardiac care, and worked with the contract cardiologists who traveled from Kalispell. Alan's schooling was periodically interrupted, and he would spend one semester in Michigan studying and another with his wife in Browning.

Alan adopted one of the stray reservation dogs. Buster was a ninety pound, "Heinz 57" variety mutt. He was pure white, and gentle. Buster would go on hikes with his masters, and then sleep soundly after that. Alan would say of Buster, "He's got some Indian blood in him."

Justine was a conscientious employee, and took her work very seriously. She went to work early and came home late. I knew this because she walked past my quarters to and from the hospital. Jonie Hind recruited her to coordinate the cardiac clinic in Browning and to work with the visiting cardiologists during their visits.

"I don't have proper nursing support, and I have to do all the paperwork myself," she said.

"The nurse I do have really doesn't know enough about cardiology to be very much help. Jonie said I would get more support than I am getting," she said.

After months of overwork, frustration and under appreciation at the Blackfeet Hospital, Justine decided to leave the Indian Health Service and work for one of the same cardiologists in Kalispell who was contracted to provide service to Browning. As their employee, she would travel back to Browning with them for their periodic clinics. Justine and I would quickly catch up on family matters between patients.

Justine and Alan moved from Browning to a rental house in Whitefish at the base of Big Mountain. During the two winters I was without Linda, they often invited me over for dinner, a movie or to watch our respective college teams compete on TV. The intrastate rivalry between the University of Michigan and Michigan State University is legendary. Since they were from Ann Arbor and Justine had worked for the University of Michigan Hospitals, our rivalry was fun. They lived in Whitefish my second winter, and I sometimes stayed overnight at their house. It was very convenient for skiing at Big Mountain.

Justine and Alan were avid bikers. From the time of the snows melting until the Park officially opened for the summer, Glacier National Park was for the exclusive enjoyment of the locals. In May, the three of us rode our bicycles from the west entrance of the Going-to-the-Sun Road up to an area called The Loop. The road is closed to motorized vehicular traffic until the snow melts at Logan Pass, at the Continental Divide. This date can be as late as June. It was a beautiful day and scenic bike ride.

My winter continued with skiing at Big Mountain on weekends and cross-country skiing on some evenings during the week. Linda was convinced I was out partying and carousing every night, but in truth I was not. I missed her and our life together, and filled my life with these other activities.

Most of my week nights were filled with the mundane chores of meal preparation, laundry, reading, and TV. Most Friday afternoons were spent cleaning the apartment, laundry, reading, and sometimes napping.

One beautiful Friday winter afternoon I decided to go cross-country skiing alone on the road to Two Medicine Lake. Harold and I had an agreement to let each other know where we were going skiing as a safety measure. He was still working at the pharmacy, and I called him from home to let him know where I was headed. There was no cell phone service in Glacier National Park, but I had my four-wheel drive Mountaineer. I drove further into the deep snow than I should have, and got stuck. Here I was, five miles out of East Glacier without cell phone service, stuck in the road. This was the first time I had been stuck in my SUV. A few thoughts went through my head. "What if I can't get the truck out? If I have to walk or ski, it may take me a few hours to get to East Glacier. The road ahead is closed for the winter, and there is absolutely no traffic here. I could very well be in deep trouble."

Fortunately, I was prepared and I had a snow shovel. I shoveled out a path for the wheels. I then used my floor mats for traction, and was finally able to free the SUV.

I called a worried Harold when I got home that evening.

The locals (Harold) warn that everyone who drives into the mountains during winter should have a full tank of gas, survival supplies, food, and a change of warm clothes.

I always heeded that good advice.

Montana really is the Wild, Wild West.

* * *

I only had enough accrued annual leave to spend either Christmas or New Years with Linda that year, so I flew to Texas for New Years. Flying to Texas from Montana is an all-day affair. If I left Great Falls early in the morning, I would spend the night before at the Hampton Inn, five minutes from the airport. It was a two-hour drive from Browning to Great Falls in normal weather.

The Inn had complimentary transportation on their shuttle van, and free parking for my car in their parking lot until my return. I often traveled from the Hampton Inn with the Denver air crew for my flight. We would fly from Great Falls to Denver; from there to either Dallas or Houston, and then to the Killeen/Fort Hood Regional airport where Linda would pick me up for the twenty-minute drive home to Harker Heights.

Another route was from Kalispell/Seattle/Minneapolis/Dallas/Killeen or Kalispell/Salt Lake/Dallas/Killeen.

You basically cannot get there from here easily. It was hard to leave my wife in Texas after the short holiday break. Our plan was for Linda to join me in Browning in the spring, and stay as long as the weather held up in the fall. I was turning sixty in May, and very much wanted to celebrate my birthday with Linda.

In February, I received an anguished phone call from Linda about our beloved Yorkshire terrier, Lucky. I was spending the weekend in Whitefish as usual, and her call woke me up at 1am. Crying, she said,

"Lucky is desperately ill and needs extensive surgery for his pancreatitis."

We decided not to go ahead with the surgery. It seems that Lucky's condition had been misdiagnosed, and his illness was caused by overuse of certain medications to treat the wrong problem. We finally got Lucky to the proper animal hospital, but by then, it was too late.

Lucky had been going downhill for several weeks, and I even considered taking him to the nearest veterinary college at Texas A & M two hours away from Harker Heights. Had we done that, we might have saved his life. Living in Ithaca, New York within a ten-minute drive of Cornell University's vet school spoiled us. Cornell veterinarians saved the life of Muffin, one of our Silky terriers.

Without my being present beside Linda, we made the painful decision to put Lucky down. Next to Muffin's untimely death, that was one of the saddest days of our lives. Lucky had been an affectionate, smart dog, which played well with our rescue toy poodle, Precious. He was a great swimmer, and we called him our "Yorkshire Labrador Retriever". One day, we took Lucky with us on a picnic to a lake near our Texas home. He started swimming after ducks, and he swam so far out that I nearly had to go after him. I seriously considered filing a complaint with the Texas State Board of Veterinary Medicine about Lucky's substandard care at the neighborhood vet clinic, but I did not go through with it. The process would have been too painful, and would not have brought Lucky back. I sincerely hope that vet learned from the experience to refer other sick animals to experts when they did not know the proper diagnosis and treatment.

I flew to Texas in early May for the purpose of driving Linda, our other car, and the two remaining dogs Precious and Sparky back to Browning. The one thousand- nine- hundred-mile trip was uneventful. About the only redeeming features of the government quarters in addition to being within walking distance of work were the well fenced in yards and great views of the mountains. Our dogs would at least be safe from wild animals and other stray dogs. We did observe one docile neighborhood dog climb the fence and escape his yard.

I had invited my new Montana friends to celebrate my sixtieth birthday and to meet Linda. Linda attempted to bake a birthday cake, but it came out uncooked. The I oven was an old, bottom of the line Magic Chef, and the temperature control was inaccurate. I put in a work order to repair the oven.

Word got out among the maintenance workers that my wife was from Texas, and therefore could not possibly know how to bake at altitude. Browning is at four-thousand- three-hundred feet above sea level. What these geniuses did not know was that Linda spent three years successfully cooking and baking in New Mexico at five-thousand five-hundred feet above sea level.

Instead of replacing this tired, broken unit with old style electric burners with a new stove, the I decided to pay a fortune to replace the broken thermostat instead. We ordered my birthday cake from Costco. The party took place as planned, and Linda had an opportunity to meet friends and neighbors.

She soon settled into her usual routine of beautifying our living space. Our original maintenance man managed to paint the walls white. All the interior trim and doors were unfinished bare wood. Linda varnished all the trim and interior doors, making a large improvement in the appearance of the place. The yard was large and weed-filled, needing to be dug up and reseeded. The air conditioning unit was rusted and did not work. We had a new assigned maintenance man as our original one formally retired (he worked like he was already retired when he worked). The IHS did not have the money to put in a new lawn, even though the previous occupants had a large dog that wore pathways in the yard.

Largely due to extreme winds and arid conditions, Browning is practically treeless. The only trees on the Great Plains are those along streams and creeks. There are a few hearty specimens that must have been well-cared for near a few dwellings. Linda decided we needed trees in our yard. With the requisite approval but predicted negativity of Bob Jones, we planted trees in our yard. Where did we get the trees? We reasoned that moving trees from one part of the reservation to another would be perfectly acceptable so we spent several weekends searching for wild trees on reservation lands north of Browning towards St. Mary. As it turns out, the Red Eagle Fire burned the areas where we harvested trees later that summer. We saved a few from the fire.

Our summer together was wonderful. Because of my noon departure from work on Fridays, we often left Browning as soon as I got home and changed my clothes. The car would be packed, and Linda would hand me a peanut butter and jelly sandwich as we drove out of town. Linda had never been to Idaho, and had romanticized about the place. One of our first trips out of Montana was to Coeur d'Alene. We drove across Marias Pass to Kalispell, and from there along the beautiful west shore of Flathead Lake. We headed west through the enchanting town of Paradise, Montana on the Clark Fork River before reaching the Interstate to Idaho.

CDA, as the locals refer it to, was a nice town. It was situated on a large lake with all sorts of outdoor activities available. After checking into one of the LaQuinta motels (they take dogs), I saw that the clock in our room seemed to be an hour ahead. I began to reset the clock, when I realized we were now in the Pacific Time Zone. We explored CDA, and then decided to make the short trip west to Spokane, Washington. We spent a night at another LaQuinta in Spokane, and explored their downtown river location. Of course, we also had to check out the local Costco.

Montana had no sales tax, except in resort areas of Whitefish and Big Sky where they had a resort tax of a few percent. Washington State merchants will waive their sales tax for any Montana resident who made a purchase there. We returned from that trip via another route that took us to Missoula. I enjoy visiting college campuses, and was surprised at how small the University of Montana's campus was.

We continued along the east Shore of Flathead Lake, first stopping in Polson at the southernmost point of the lake. We spent the night at the Best Western in Polson, overlooking Flathead Lake. This is the largest freshwater lake west of the Mississippi and is one of the most beautiful. High mountains on the east border it. It reminded me of a larger version of Lake Tahoe. Polson is located on the Salish Kooteny/Flathead Indian reservation. It was also considered to be Montana's "banana belt", due to its moderate climate. The area has become a booming region of second homes from people from Missoula and elsewhere.

When we were not traveling out of state, we spent a fair amount of time looking at real estate in the Flathead Valley. Our house in New Mexico finally sold in May, right after my birthday. We used the equity in that home to pay off the subprime mortgage on the Texas home. This subsequently turned out to be one of Linda's best ideas, given the current U.S. housing situation. I had no other job prospects at this time, and we reasoned that we would purchase a primary residence somewhere in the Flathead Valley. I would move into a smaller apartment in Browning, commute during the week like Harold, and we would figure out some place for Linda to go to during the cold winter months.

We worked with a realtor from Coldwell Banker in Whitefish. She lived in a nice house with her family on a choice lakefront location on Whitefish Lake. Her husband was from Aspen, Colorado having moved there as general manager of the Aspen Mountain Ski Company to take a similar position at Big Mountain. He left Big Mountain but he and the family remained in Whitefish.

The realtor was a pleasant woman, but definitely traveled in the elite circles of Whitefish society. Before the current housing slump, this was one of the hottest housing markets in the U.S. Many wealthy people from California and other places like an old Adirondack millionaire friend bought expensive properties in Whitefish and Bigfork, on Flathead Lake. Our realtor never showed us a place that was really affordable.

We then focused our search in Columbia Falls, which was the blue-collar suburb of Kalispell. It is the site of the big Plum Creek Paper Mill, and is closer to Browning. One day we were driving through a neighborhood in Columbia Falls, and we saw several lots in a row for sale on the banks of the Flathead River. We had just enough cash left after paying off Texas to purchase a lot, and then build our Montana dream house on it.

We really liked one lot that was one-and-a-half acres situated on the high bank of the Flathead River. "We could build steps down to the river so you could use your kayak," Linda said.

"There is public river access right next to this parcel," I replied.

We began to design our dream house, determining its orientation on the lot, and what trees we'd have to remove along the river bank to improve the view. After spending an afternoon exploring the parcel, we decided to go back to the real estate office and make a purchase offer.

It turned out that the "For Sale" sign was on the wrong parcel, and the one we were interested in was not for sale. This ultimately resulted in our not tying up one-hundred-fifty-thousand dollars cash for a lot in Columbia Falls, Montana.

Another highlighted trip over the July fourth holiday was to the Canadian Rockies. We drove north through Waterton Lakes National Park, Alberta through a beautiful area west of Calgary. From there we drove to the town of Banff. Canada had a holiday that weekend, and we enjoyed watching a parade and fireworks at night. We found Banff to be charming. We continued west and stopped at the magnificent Columbia Ice Fields. We did not actually hike to the glacier, but spent time on the moraine field before it. This gem of nature is expected to be another casualty of global warming in the near future.

There were markers showing the retreat of the glacier over the last hundred or so years.

We continued west through some of the most spectacular mountain scenery I have ever seen, and of course had to spend time at Lake Louise. This is one of the famous World Heritage Sites. It is so spectacular that this designation transcends even the National Park or Wilderness title.

We had brunch at the fabled Lake Louise Lodge, where rooms started at six-hundred- dollars a night (and they don't allow dogs). We hiked along the lake, taking in the breathtaking scenery. Our final destination was Jasper National Park, where we ended that day. We were disappointed with our visit, finding high prices for everything and substandard accommodations. We did not spend time hiking there or exploring that Park due to our short time and great distance from there back to Browning.

July was also the month for Indian Days. This event showcases the Blackfeet at their finest. All year long, the native women work on lavish native costumes ornately decorated with fancy beadwork and feathers just for this week-long festival. Locals and visiting Indians alike set up teepees and other tents at the local campground. The teepees are set up like their ancestral ones, with families like the Makes Cold Weather storing the teepee poles from one year to the next.

An unwritten code exists between families where the choice camping spots are reserved for the tribal elders and councilmen. Plains Indians traveled to Browning from other tribes to participate in the dancing and to set up tables of their wares for sale. The Blackfeet dancers, both men and women, were quite athletic and well-choreographed. The dances were intricate and colorful. Indian drums beat well into the wee hours of the morning, as young Indians performed their annual ritual of "Teepee Creeping". Nine months later, there was a baby boom in Browning. I spent Indian Days of my final summer with my pharmacy friends. I knew I was beginning to be accepted when one of the Native physical therapists asked me, "How were your Indian Days?"

I doubt I will ever be asked that question again as long as I live.

Tuesday evenings were Craft Night in the hospital loop area. Primarily lead by Jonie Hind, the women gathered at someone's quarters to do craft projects. Linda had mixed feelings about the group, but she went most Tuesdays. She showed the women how to make decorative purses. On one night, Jonie declared a women's hiking night. The group planned to hike to St. Mary Falls in the Park. It rained, so they ended up eating slices of berry pies at the well-known Park Café in St. Mary. The Café motto was, "Pie For Strength." Linda enjoyed the evening.

There was a group of people living in Montana called Hutterites. They are similar to the Amish, but lived on large mechanized ranches. Jacob Hutter who immigrated to Montana from Austria many years ago founded the sect. They lived on ranches as large as thirty-thousand acres and raised hogs, cattle, and poultry. They lived as family units in neat houses they built, and they ate together in one large communal dining room. They prayed together in their church. The women only had an eighth-grade education, as more education was not considered worthwhile for these women.

Harold knew several of the men through his farming connections, and arranged a visit for a group from the hospital. Pharmacy students joined Linda, Harold, I and another neighbor as we visited a Hutterite colony near Cut Bank. Harold said, "We've got to stop for some beer in Cut Bank. It's the price of admission to the colony."

Our hosts showed us around the property. Their kitchen, slaughter house and farming operations were the cleanest I have ever seen. One could literally eat off the kitchen floor. The

Hutterite women were shy, and dressed in their characteristic long dresses. The men were bearded, wore suspenders, cowboy hats and boots. They were savvy businessmen, who also sold their products to local markets. Harold did business with them for his farming activities.

On Fridays, they would come to Browning to sell chickens, produce, eggs, and fresh baked bread out of their truck. They exported their hog products to countries like Japan. Once the colony reached one-hundred-twenty-five individuals, the elders would seek another parcel of land to set up another colony. This was not a democratic process, and people were assigned to move to the new colony.

* * *

It was impossible to ignore the abandoned and starving dogs roaming around Browning. As a sovereign nation, there was no SPCA nor animal shelter, nor formal neutering program on the Blackfeet reservation. Cruelty to animals was not a crime on an Indian reservation. Our next-door neighbor, a nurse, had organized voluntary vet services in the past, but there were never enough tribal funds available to continue the neutering program. The local veterinarian, a native Blackfeet, did what she could to provide pro-bono treatment and placement for abandoned dogs and cats.

Linda's morning routine was to drive to the local BIA office in Browning, across from the town's parking compound. Several feral dogs lived under the vehicles and in adjacent abandoned buildings. She took the extra dried dog food we had and placed plates of the food on the ground. These dogs were starving, but so fearful of humans they would not approach her. She would slowly back away from the plates, and then the dogs would eat the food. These animals were flea infested, mangy, and severely undernourished. They had probably been abused as well, hence their fear of her.

Some dogs would come and go, but two regulars Linda named "Summer" and "Hyena". She fed them during the week, but they were left to fend for themselves when we left for the weekend trips. Their health improved under Linda's hands-off care, but she could never approach them. They learned to respond to her distinctive whistle as she set down the food bowls. We almost adopted two res dogs ourselves. One we called "Jake" was a large short-haired mutt. It was hot and he was thirsty, so we kept him in the shaded yard for a day and gave him some food and water. We decided that he and Sparky would not get along, so we let him wander off. We did ask neighbors if anyone wanted him.

We came even closer to adoption of a very smart Border collie mix we named "Montana". We took this dog to the local vet for shots. We found him near the time we were leaving to return to Texas. Again, we felt Sparky and he would not get along. I gave Montana to Karen Green who said her grandson wanted a dog.

The Blackfeet have little regard for man's best friend. Linda and I learned at the Museum of the Plains Indians that dogs played a big role in the history of the Blackfeet. They served as beasts of burden long before the Spanish introduced horses, hauling shelter materials and other supplies on specially made carriers between encampments. We could not understand the callus mistreatment and neglect of dogs that was so prevalent on the modern reservation.

When I returned to Browning from driving Linda back to Texas for what was to be my final year, I asked Karen and her husband about Montana.

"How's Montana doing?'

I thought the dog would make a good companion for me if Karen's family did not want him any more. We would deal with

Sparky's adjustment at another time and Sparky was getting older. Karen's husband told me,

"A lady from Cut Bank stole him from the back yard and took him away."

When I pressed him for details, it was obvious this was clearly a fabricated story and I never believed a word of it. Karen told me of frequent Grizzly sightings in her back yard, which borders the Park.

I hoped the poor dog wasn't eaten.

I placed missing dog pictures (we did take them of Montana) in the Post Office in East Glacier, but I never heard another thing about that animal. I even called the local vet and asked her to call me if the dog surfaced again in her office.

Our last big trip prior to Linda's return to Texas was to visit friends near Sun Valley, Idaho. The recently retired doctor was the director of the chronic pain clinic who retired earlier that summer. He and his wife had become friends, as they were neighbors in Browning. His wife joined the Young and Restless ski club that previous winter on one trip to Isaac Walton. They had owned a home near Ketchum, Idaho for a number of years; planning to retire there eventually.

They invited us to visit, which we did over the Labor Day weekend. We stopped at the Patagonia Outlet store in Dillon, Montana on the way to Idaho. I purchased a few items at a fraction of their regular cost during their annual Labor Day sale. Patagonia apparel was normally expensive, and the brand was mockingly referred to as "Patagucci". We also stopped at an opal mine in Idaho just south of the Montana border. We did not have time to collect there, but Linda bought a few items. I bought her a nice finished opal necklace. We also stopped at the Craters of the Moon National Monument to add that destination to our National Parks Passbook.

Soon after Linda and I married, I introduced her to our spectacular National Park system. We took many trips west and even to Alaska and Hawaii. Linda bought a National Parks Passbook on our first trip. We have our own little hobby of collecting date stamps at National Parks and National Monuments, and bring the book with us on every trip we take in case we come across a lesser-known National Monument. Linda is our official "book stamper". We have stamps from Hawaii; Haleakala Volcano National Park on Maui, and several parks in Alaska. Of course, we have a number of stamps for Glacier. I was a volunteer at the Petroglyph National Monument in Albuquerque until the Covid pandemic.

I recommend all of you buy and use one of these books.

We arrived at five pm just after the Visitor Center closed. We drove around the landscape briefly. Linda stamped our book while the Craters of the Moon Visitor Center was open on the way home. Finally, we arrived at Guy and Josie's near twilight. Guy was an avid fly fisherman, and his home was perfect for the occasion. He would walk out his back door, through a field, and cast a line into the river behind the house. Josie had found her niche in the local art community. They were both avid cyclists and the area was perfect for riding. They became our role model for retirement.

Linda had always wanted to visit Sun Valley, so after breakfast, Guy and Josie drove us to that area. We spent some time at a local flea market outside of Ketchum, and then explored Sun Valley. There was an auto auction with some very expensive cars, fitting for upscale Sun Valley. Linda and I were not impressed with that area and quickly crossed it off our list as a possible place to retire.

After lunch, we left Guy and Josie and drove to Boise. We traveled through the mountains to Stanley and from there to Boise. The Sawtooth Mountains were impressive, but the arduous drive through switchback turns was tiring and endless. We finally arrived at our downtown hotel around dinner time. I had visited Boise in 1972 in my "other life", but remembered little of that trip. Boise reminded us both of Syracuse, New York. We strolled around the capitol area and dined at the hotel restaurant. The valley was filled with smoke from the many wildfires that had plagued the region over that summer.

The lowest point in our otherwise wonderful summer was the death of our beloved rescue poodle, Precious. Linda found Precious wandering on the streets of Ithaca scrounging for bugs. She was emaciated, flea-infested, and near death. We took her to our vet and she recovered well. She was a smart and affectionate companion. The vet thought she was about seven or eight years old at the time. She got along well with Sparky and Lucky, but was at times at odds with our other female Silky Terrier, Muffin.

One summer night in Browning, we were awakened by the sounds of Precious yelping in pain. We initially thought she was having bad dreams. We took her to the local vet clinic outside of Browning. The vet thought that Precious was having heart problems-she was about fourteen years old. Per the doctor's suggestion, I injected saline solution subcutaneously into Precious's neck (you may recall my previous DVM license). This only provided temporary relief. She continued to have these heart seizures. Finally, on a Saturday after several more episodes, we felt it was time to put her out of her obvious pain and misery.

We drove Precious to a vet clinic in Kalispell, and they euthanized her that morning. I was too distraught to be in the exam room for the lethal injection, but Linda stood by her side comforting her to the end. Precious is buried behind Quarters number twelve in Browning under a tree we planted in her memory.

We began to make plans to return Linda to Texas, but we decided to acquire another vehicle to make the trip. Our 2006

Toyota Avalon was a great car, but it actually had less trunk room than Linda's 1997 Avalon. We were interested in looking into hybrid vehicles. We also needed an SUV to eventually replace the aging and gas guzzling Mountaineer. The only 2007 hybrid SUV's available were the Toyota Highlander and the Ford Escape/Mercury Mariner models.

We had heard that there would be a 2008 Chevy Tahoe hybrid in 2008, but we could not wait for that. Since Montana had no sales tax, it was a great place to purchase a big-ticket item such as an SUV.

We ordered our 2007 Highlander hybrid from City Toyota in Great Falls. We did not get a great deal, but we also did not pay full sticker either. The Toyota dealership in Kalispell wanted to charge us full sticker price plus another thousand-dollar premium for the new hybrid. Our new vehicle was ready in mid-September, and we picked it up in Great Falls. The IRS was giving tax incentives that year to those who purchased hybrid vehicles, and we just made the cutoff of September thirtieth.

We made one trip in the Highlander over the Going-to-the Sun Road with our friends, Justine and Alan. We also made a shorter trip in that car to Bigfork for dinner with Harold and Pam. It was October, and time for us to drive back to Texas.

Linda made it crystal clear that she would never set foot in Browning again. In spite of our wonderful summer, she could never again live in such a drug infested, animal cruelty-plagued, impoverished, and corrupt place. This was a great motivation to find another job elsewhere, since I wanted to remain married to Linda.

Our trip back was long and uneventful. The Highlander averaged twenty-four and a half mpg highway. Not that impressive compared to today's technology.

I flew back to Great Falls for what I hoped would be my final months in Browning. I was alone again, with both the Avalon and Mountaineer for my use. The Mountaineer was a perfect Montana vehicle, and were it not for the poor gas mileage, we would have kept it. My plans were to keep it for the winter and sell it in the spring/summer. The Avalon barely fit in the tight one car garage, with about two inches of clearance to close the garage door. Most of the time I drove the Mountaineer except in good weather when I drove the Avalon to keep the battery charged. In May, I purchased a season pass for Big Mountain for the next ski season for four-hundred-seventy-five dollars. I figured that if another job came my way before the season, I could get a refund. For those readers who do not ski, a season's pass allows one to ski any day the area is open. In other words, you get paid to ski as much as possible. I skied twenty-one days that season, making my daily cost for skiing just under twenty three dollars. A full price adult ticket was fifty-two dollars per day. The added convenience of not having to stand in line to purchase a daily ticket, and the luxury of leaving the mountain in bad weather without guilt was also more than worth the initial cost.

Second and Final Winter without Linda

I flew back to Montana in October after driving Linda and Sparky back to Harker Heights in our new Highlander. I returned to my usual routine of working during the week and amusing myself on weekends. Sparky was growing old-his hearing was gone and his eyesight was failing. Linda was actively searching for replacement dogs, as we knew Sparky would not last much longer. By searching the Internet, she came across a breed of dogs called Havanese. This was a relatively new breed in the U.S., although more popular in Germany and Canada. She began an email correspondence with a breeder in Hague, Saskatchewan. I had recently opened a new MasterCard account where using the card for purchases would benefit my alma mater, Michigan State University.

Linda placed an order for two Havanese puppies for a total of sixteen-hundred dollars each. The breeder charged my new MasterCard the full amount of thirty-two hundred dollars, with an approximate shipping date of eight weeks hence. After placing the order, Linda did some further research about the breed on Cornell University's vet school website. She was dismayed to find that this breed was known to have significant health problems.

Having suffered through Precious and Lucky's problems, she did not wish to go through that agony again. Linda canceled the order less than forty-eight hours after she placed it and eight weeks prior to shipping. The breeder initially agreed to refund the entire amount but then recanted and said she would issue the refund only after reselling the puppies.

We protested the charge, and MasterCard initially reversed the entire amount while they investigated. I closed the account immediately after they reversed the charge. The situation between Linda and the breeder became ugly, with her accusing Linda of trying to become a puppy mill for this breed. We filed a complaint with the Better Business Bureau in Canada. She finally agreed to settle the account for a deposit fee of Nine hundred forty-six dollars. After checking her website again, Linda believed that she had already sold these two puppies, thus she was essentially stealing nearly a thousand dollars from us for no product or merchandise-at no cost to her.

One of the painful lessons we learned from this was that credit card companies did not have the same policies for consumer protection. MasterCard was the most merchant friendly, stating that they did not have the authority to interfere with a merchant's right to set their own refund policies. There was no mention of a deposit requirement, nor was there any description of a refund policy on the breeder's website. Visa was more consumer-friendly, with American Express offering the best consumer protection policy of the major credit card companies at that time. Without my knowledge or permission, MasterCard opened a new account and transferred the nine hundred forty-six-dollar balance to it.

Bank of America oversaw MasterCard, and they continued to hound me for payment. We hired our attorney in Kalispell to write a letter to Bank of America- to no avail. I contacted Michigan State University to notify them regarding my troubles. I filed complaints with the Internet Fraud Bureau, the Comptroller of the Currency, and Montana Senator Max Baucus. I also contacted the local office of the Royal Canadian Mounted Police in Hague to investigate this as a criminal matter. I was able to negotiate with Bank of America to split the difference- the time and agony of fighting this was wearing me down. The following is a letter to a senior staffer with Bank of America:

> **I have received your letter of January 24, 2008 regarding my account ending in 0289.**
>
> **Enclosed please find a check for the amount of $463.40 to satisfy the entire debt on this**
>
> **Account per our telephone agreement of January 22, 2008. I appreciate your efforts in protecting my valuable credit rating by notifying the credit agencies, and in eliminating the interest and penalty charges.**
>
> **In addition to submitting this payment in full to satisfy the outstanding balance on this account, I am requesting the following actions from MasterCard:**
>
> **1. Please provide a letter acknowledging total relief of my liability of this disputed charge.**

2. Please provide assurances that neither this account, my original Michigan State University account, nor another MasterCard account be opened or ever be used or charged in the future without my knowledge and expressed written consent.

3. Please notify your Phoenix office and FIA Card Services, N.A. to cease their harassing telephone calls and all threatening correspondence regarding this account.

I am settling this matter in the agreed upon manner to put an end to this nightmare that began in November 2006, not because I believe the vendor is legally entitled to the money. I strongly feel that MasterCard needs to provide better protection for the consumer while still allowing honest merchants to reveal up front their clearly stated return and cancelation policies to potential customers. Legitimate businesses do not change these policies on a whim or in retaliation for a justified complaint for the purpose of stealing money from customers.

I recognize you are in a business for profit. Nevertheless, not everyone with a credit card terminal and bank account represents a legitimate business worthy of the privilege of accepting credit cards. MasterCard should never allow itself to be placed in a position to support the questionable or blatantly unlawful business practices of their clients under the ruse of "policies that best suit their business needs." I suggest that MasterCard should at the very least check with the Better Business Bureau (in Canada in this instance) or with State's Attorney General's Office for any previous or existing consumer complaints involving the prospective merchant prior to accepting them as a new client. There should also be a mechanism to remove unscrupulous businesses from the MasterCard program.

After all, isn't customer satisfaction "Priceless"?

* * *

The bank responded by letter accepting my check and agreeing to my terms.

Linda and I learned valuable lessons from this. There is little the U.S. can do to protect its citizens against illegal transactions that transpire outside the United States. We will certainly become aware of cancelation, refund, and deposit requirements in the future.

* * *

Harold had often expressed his respect for my work and me and was fascinated with my descriptions of some of the surgical procedures I performed. As director of the pharmacy education program in Browning, he was also interested in having pharmacy students observe surgery. I'd had medical, nursing, and PA students observe in some of my cases and I did not see any reason why pharmacy students could not be included. There is a good deal of pharmacy going on in the OR by the anesthesia providers, and Harold and I felt it would be good for them to see the delivery end of their work.

As Chairman of the Surgical Committee, in conjunction with the Head OR nurse, we established a program to educate any who desired to observe in surgery. This policy was necessary to assure sterility of the surgical field. I received permission from one patient to have Harold and students observe her surgery. I gave Harold about a five-minute crash course in OR protocol and proper dress as we entered the operating room.

I had been performing podiatric surgery for thirty years. I have worked with all calibers of assistants, with Terry Valentino of Fort Hood being the Gold Standard. Browning had two old hens (I was older than both of them) who complained constantly about their aches and pains while lifting the patient's leg (she was thin). Their quality of care came close to the bottom tier of those I had worked with previously. I am constantly amazed at how health care professionals can so easily be distracted from their purpose of why they are there: It should always be about the patient, and nothing else really matters.

Surgical masks hide facial expressions, but Harold knew me well enough to know I was not happy. After I made the first incision of a multiple incision foot surgery, the power saw failed. While I was waiting for the old hens to find another working saw, I made the second incision. Harold was astounded that I would do this before I knew I had another working saw. This surgery was being done with the use of a tourniquet and therefore I did not wish to waste valuable tourniquet time while the women bitched and argued about the equipment.

Harold was a farmer and is used to doing things with his hands. As he began to reach over towards the sterile field with his bare hands to help out, I said, "Harold, don't touch anything!"

The surgery went well after the other saw was located, as I knew it would be. Harold thought that the whole experience was pretty cool, and afterwards he expressed this to Pam and everybody else who would listen.

Wrong site surgery was more of a problem in the past until recently. Now, before every surgical case, surgeons nationwide are required to go through a "time out" process with the operating room staff.

The process goes something like this: The surgeon will actually sign their initials using a purple skin marker adjacent to the operative site while the patient is in the holding area. After the patient is wheeled into the operating room, the circulating nurse will ask the patient, "What is your name and social security number?"

After the patient identifies himself, the nurse will say out loud to all members of the team, "This is Rick Jones, and he is going to have a bunionectomy on his left foot, does everyone agree?"

I guess it's similar to a wedding ceremony where the guests are asked if anyone objects to the pending marriage. After agreement is reached, the operation begins. The origin of this helpful process originated from incident years ago at a Tampa hospital. A busy surgeon swept into the operating room where a patient's leg was already prepped and draped for surgery. The doctor proceeded to amputate the leg.

It was the wrong one.

It seems that this particular diabetic patient required both leg amputations eventually, but that glaring medical error was the seminal event in instituting the "time out" procedure around the country. I invented my own phrase to describe this activity,

"We don't always operate on the right foot but we always do the correct one."

During my last spring in Montana, my friends and I were looking for a way to keep up our fitness from the winter's skiing. Beginning sometime in April, Harold, another contract pharmacist and I would go for bicycle rides beginning at 6:30am before work. We would ride for thirty minutes around the housing developments in Browning dodging stray dogs, logging trucks and occasional carcasses of dead dogs.

With no trees growing on the plains, we had an unobstructed view of sunlight brightly shining on the Front Range of the Rockies into Glacier National Park. I would also ride my bike after work, alone or with friends.

The scenery always reminded me of the song, "America the Beautiful". I used to hum it to myself as I rode my bike. Katharine

Lee Bates wrote the lyrics to this song in 1893 after an inspiring trip to the top of Pikes Peak in Colorado.

I believe she would have been equally inspired had she visited Glacier National Park instead.

Browning was without a doubt the windiest place I have ever lived. Ranches on the outskirts of town were fenced in with barbed wire. There were thousands of white plastic shopping bags from the world's largest retailer caught in every fence, flapping in the stiff breezes. A trip from Browning to Walmart was a full day's affair, with the nearest stores either two hours south in Great Falls, or two hours west in Kalispell. A trip to Walmart was a common reason given for patients missing appointments in my clinic. Other trash, beer bottles and cans from the night before and other flotsam were strewn over wide areas, in sharp contrast to the surrounding spectacular scenery.

During the summer months, it would stay light until nearly 11 pm due to the northern latitude of Montana. That left several hours of good daylight after work for outdoor activities. One of my favorite sports was taking my kayak into Glacier Park after work. One night, the pharmacy crew had a picnic on the shores of Two Medicine Lake. Due to their work schedules, it did not begin until after 8 pm. I let Gary Barker's teenage son try out my boat. He paddled out of sight. As it got darker, we were beginning to worry about him. Gary said, "I hope he doesn't get lost."

I was annoyed because I did not have a chance to paddle my own boat again on this beautiful evening. Finally, Gary said, "I'd better see if I can find him."

Gary hiked along the shore of the lake as far as he could. Finally, his son came paddling back around the point as darkness set in. I asked Gary's permission to talk to his son, and he said, "Sure, go ahead."

I was annoyed, and I said, "Did you lose track of time?" Did you give any thought that people might be worried about you?" Did you think I might want to paddle my own boat?"

He got the message.

I also enjoyed kayaking on Swift Current Lake and St. Mary Lake, both in the Park. I had never paddled in more scenic places. On one occasion as I was kayaking alone, I was startled by the slap of a beaver's tail on the surface of Two Medicine Lake. The beaver dove, swam under my boat, and slapped his tail again. I cleared the area per its insistent request.

As I was sorting out my mail from a daily trip to the Browning Post Office, I glanced at a letter from the Medicare office in Binghamton, New York. At first glance, I couldn't imagine what they were contacting me for. I also wondered how they got my current address, after moving so many times since leaving Ithaca.

Big Brother is watching.

I opened the letter and was stunned by its content.

They were demanding a $20,000 payment relating to the results of their audit some six years earlier! The payment was due in thirty days with a check made out to the "United States Treasury." The letter went on to say something like this in government speak, "Don't even think about defaulting, we know where you live and work."

When they left my office in Ithaca and said it would be "some time" before I heard from them, I had no idea they meant six years.

I had the right to a formal hearing to address their concerns, and a special judge would decide the result of the hearing. The problem was I had no direct access to the patient files, and I was living over two thousand miles from Ithaca, New York.

I immediately contacted my trusted attorney in Buffalo, New York who had previously handled other matters for me when I lived in that state, and he agreed to represent me.

I called my old office to request copies of the old chart notes, and the current owner charged me fifty dollars for the service. I was not happy, but I had to pay his fee to receive the records. Meanwhile, I kept asking my attorney about a statute of limitations. Surely Medicare should not be permitted to pursue matters such as this forever, could they?

I spent hours reviewing the pertinent medical records and recalling the patient's problems. This many years later, I was having difficulty placing names and faces together.

I arranged the hearing for a Friday afternoon when I was off work. It was a three-way telephone conference between me in Browning, my attorney in Buffalo, and the hearing officer in Binghamton. Of course, we had to consider the two-hour time zone difference between Montana and New York. I went through each and every of the twenty charts to justify my treatment and billing to Medicare for these services. The process was tedious, time consuming and onerous.

Less than six years later (about a month less), I received the judge's decision.

He ruled that Medicare had exceeded the three-year statute of limitations, and they were not entitled to collect a cent. The exercise of a formal hearing was moot based strictly on the time issue. I wish I had known that before all the hassle.

For a $2,000 legal fee, I was allowed to keep my original $20,000.

Score one for the little guy.

* * *

During one of my frequent visits to Harold and Pam's in the spring, I found Harold out in the fields plowing for the new wheat crop. He saw me and drove over in his John Deere tractor.

"Evan, have you ever plowed a field before?"

"No, I'm really a city boy."

"Climb aboard."

I climbed into this giant $100,000 plus behemoth of a tractor, and Harold drove us back out to the fields his father and grandfather plowed before him.

"This machine has air conditioning and even a radio," he said.

I looked out the back of the cab at the large row of plow blades, thinking, "This was a far cry from the horse drawn plows of yesteryear."

Harold finished plowing that forty-acre field in no time.

During ski season, after I finished skiing for the day at Big Mountain, I would often visit Harold and Pam.

Harold was trying to finish the tack room for Pam's tack, and I helped him.

"Evan, give me a hand with the insulation."

I held the ladder and helped him insulate the room.

Harold also gave me an extensive education about various saddles, but I'm afraid I forgot most of it. He was a rodeo rider in his younger years, and knew a great deal about that subject.

Pam said to Harold, "Are you ever going to finish my tack room?"

Harold was easily distracted, and had many projects going on at the same time.

The room was still not finished when I left Montana.

The last long weekend of the summer, Labor Day arrived. I was homeless and without my car. Harold invited me to spend the weekend with him at his farm in the Flathead Valley, and to help him with the wheat crop. Pam was away on an Alaskan cruise, assisting a disabled friend. The deal was I would work for room and board for the weekend. Montana wheat was of the finest quality, and harvesting was done around Labor Day.

Wheat farmers must quickly harvest the crop before rain falls which increases the moisture content of the wheat. Harold hired a friend with a combine to harvest his two hundred acres. The yield averaged sixty to ninety bushels per acre. The separated wheat kernels were conveyed into waiting open trucks to be driven to the grain elevators in Kalispell. Harold kept a silo full of grain as seed for next year's crops. I helped him with that task, helped fix flat tires on his pivots (irrigation rigs), and did most of the cooking for the weekend.

On Labor Day, we drove the loaded trucks to the elevators for weighing and dumping. I drove a 1972 International Harvester truck, that Harold dubbed the "Interceptor", due to its distinctive black and white markings. It had no seat belts, and had dubious brakes, but the trip was not far. As I drove the truck onto the scales, the elevator operators measured the moisture content of the wheat. If the level was over thirteen-and-a-half percent they could not accept the load. Fortunately, Harold's wheat met the standard, and was dumped into the elevator containers. He received a receipt for a prearranged price per bushel derived from futures pricing. I never really understood the business aspect of wheat farming. I asked Harold, "Do you actually make money at this, or is it just a hobby?"

He answered, "I usually cover my expenses and sometimes make a little more depending on the going price of wheat, but it's really a way of life here."

I never was able to sort out the truth, but it was probably somewhere in all of the above. After weighing the truck, I was asked to get out subtracting my weight. Whenever anyone asks how much I weigh, I answer, "Three bushels of wheat."

Later that fall, Harold tipped over one of his old grain trucks while avoiding certain to be fatal crash into a lady's small car. He and the lady were unhurt, but he lost some valuable grain and a truck windshield.

His brakes failed.

Farming is a dangerous occupation under the best of circumstances, but all the more so with old, poorly maintained equipment.

I did learn to appreciate the efforts that go into harvesting wheat, and smile as I recall my farmers weekend whenever I bite into a piece of bread.

After moving to Mississippi, we found a wonderful bakery in Jackson. The owner noticed my Montana license plates, and said, "Are you from Montana?"

"I just moved from there."

"My wheat comes from Montana."

"What part?"

"I get my wheat from Havre."

"That's not too far from Browning where I just moved from." I said.

The Great Harvest Bread Company is actually a franchise, headquartered in Great Falls, Montana. How coincidental. I saw another Great Harvest store in East Lansing, Michigan during a trip back to Michigan State.

Some years before I arrived in Browning, Harold was president of the Montana Mint Growers Association. Harold and his late brother grew mint on the same land he later grew wheat. The brothers designed and built a mint still on their property. Harold, a pharmacist by training, was ideally suited for this business. Mint plants were harvested at the proper time, and then were transferred to the still where the valuable mint oil was extracted and purified from the crop.

The buyers of mint oil were large companies such as Wrigley gum, Life Saver and others. Harold told me that the mint oil from Montana was of the highest quality, but that the candy and confection manufacturers were able to use the inferior but cheaper foreign mint. This signaled the end of the mint business in the Flathead Valley.

I saw Harold's still before it was dismantled and sold to a California mint grower. With my chemistry background, I could appreciate the process and the still's efficient design. During the distillation process, Harold said, "The Valley used to be filled with the pleasant aroma of mint during processing season."

I briefly considered studying natural product chemistry in graduate school, but chose biochemistry instead. The haze one often sees over distant vistas of forests during the heat of summer (Great Smoky Mountains) is caused by natural products emitted by trees called terpenes (turpentine). Unless it's smoke from a wildfire.

On the Tuesday after Labor Day, Harold drove us back to Browning. He normally had Mondays off.

Harold invited me to his Kalispell home for my final weekend in Montana. I wanted to go, but Linda insisted I stay in Browning to rest up for the rigors of the pending move. On that Friday after work, I walked back to Harold's place near the hospital and began a quiet weekend alone of reading, rest and reflection. Harold had no TV at his quarters, but I did wander down to the pharmacy students' trailer to watch a college football game on Saturday. It was the most peaceful weekend I'd ever had.

Harold arrived back to work on Tuesday morning. I stayed at his place that last night and arranged to be picked up by a neighbor at 3:30am the next morning for a ride back to Kalispell and the airport. Harold and I said our sad goodbyes and I arrived in Texas later that same evening.

During one leg of the flight back to Texas, I had a voice mail message on my cell phone that was turned off during the flight. It was from the HR clerk in Jackson who was handling my paperwork, it said, "This is Maria from the Jackson VA, please call me as soon as possible."

I called her at the airport in Dallas. She said, "Dr. Meltzer, I'm formally offering you this job at the agreed upon salary, do you accept?"

"I'm on my way, so I guess the answer is yes."

Chapter Five

Is it Hampton, Jackson, or San Diego?

East Coast, West Coast All Around the Town

Ever since I learned that my Fort Hood contracting job would end in a year, I developed the daily habit of looking at the government websites for job postings in my field. I decided to stay with the government as a full-time employee until retirement for the health care and other retirement benefits. I had been without personal health insurance for several years, and as a veteran myself I began to rely on the VA for my healthcare. This works ok if you live near a VA facility. In the spring of 2005, the only available government posted job in my field was on the Blackfeet Reservation in Montana. While I enjoyed my time in Montana, I knew from day one that this would not be my final government job.

My workdays in Browning began with getting a complementary cup of coffee from the hospital kitchen and sitting down at my computer before patients arrived (the nearest Starbucks was either two hours south or west of Browning). I would then check in by phone with my wife in Texas, and proceed to look at podiatry job postings on the USAJOBS website. My computer keyboard had wear marks on the letters, P O D I A T R I S T. After a year of treating Native Americans, I decided I would rather return to treating my fellow veterans in a suitable location where Linda and I could live together again.

My search yielded two VA podiatry jobs on the USAJOBS website; one in Hampton, Virginia and the other in Jackson, Mississippi.

I applied for both.

We visited the Hampton area just prior to leaving for New Mexico, but we had never been to Mississippi. I subsequently received phone calls from Jackson inquiring if I was still interested in the position, and I said yes. I completed a telephone interview with three staff members of the Surgical Service at the G. V. (Sonny) Montgomery VA Medical Center in Jackson. I had not heard a word from Hampton at that point. Jackson invited me for a site visit, and all expenses were paid for this June trip. At the end of the visit which I thought was still a job interview, I was offered the position. Things progress in an orderly but ponderous manner in hiring a doctor as a VA employee. The process often takes months. In August, I was two days away from boarding a plane in Montana for a house-hunting trip to Jackson when I received a call from the podiatrist at the Hampton VA. He asked, "Are you interested in participating in a telephone interview?"

"Yes."

The interview was Thursday. On Friday, the podiatrist called me back and said, "You are my first choice, but Human Resources has to make the formal offer."

I replied, "I am already in process for the Jackson job, but would prefer Hampton if that could be arranged."

I also asked, "What took you so long to get in touch?"

He said, "The HR (read "Human Roadblock") department here required me to interview all candidates and rank them. Since I had twenty applicants, this took awhile and you were my last interview."

I guess he saved the best for last!

On Saturday I boarded a plane in Great Falls, Montana to meet my wife for the trip from our home in Harker Heights, Texas to Jackson for a government-paid house-hunting trip. Monday and Tuesday were spent in Texas on the phone with the Chief of Surgery at Hampton and various members of their HR department. After a series of frustrating calls, Hampton HR decided I was too far along in the process at Jackson for them to bring me on board at their facility. Linda and I wasted two precious days of house hunting, and we finally flew to Jackson on Wednesday.

While all of this activity was going on, there was another job prospect looming in the background. I received a call from a friend and podiatry school classmate, Dr. Jeff Karn. Jeff has been practicing in San Diego since completing his residency, and was aware of a job opening at the San Diego VA. The job had not been posted yet on the USAJOBS website, but he put me in touch with the Chief of Podiatry at that facility. Jeff had never practiced in the government system, so he was not familiar with the protocols and procedures in that environment. He encouraged me to travel to San Diego at my own expense for an interview as soon as possible.

The Chief there seemed to be a kindred spirit when I first spoke with him on the phone, and we seemed to get along well. He said, "Do you cut toenails?"

"Whatever the job requires," I replied.

He responded with a jolly laugh.

We were the same age, and he was a retired Navy podiatrist and was Chief of Podiatry at the San Diego VA. The odd thing was that he acted as if this were his own private practice. He believed he could advertise for, interview and hire anyone he pleased without regard to the strict guidelines of government HR departments. He also seemed fixated on pay and moving benefits, over which he had absolutely no authority.

I flew out of Great Falls through Salt Lake City on a Monday afternoon and landed late that evening in San Diego. I spent the night with Jeff and his wife, both of whom I had not seen in many years. We stayed up until the wee hours catching up. My interview was at 11am on Tuesday.

My modus operandi has always been to befriend secretaries and administrative assistants. While waiting for the Chief, the Surgical Service secretary and I had a nice conversation. We had previously visited on the phone to set up the interview.

"You seem very busy," I said.

"Yes, I have to take care of all our residents as well as our Attending Staff."

"You appear to do it quite efficiently."

She asked me, "I'm leaving for lunch now, would you care to join me?"

"Fine," I replied, and we went to the VA Canteen for a sandwich.

At lunch I learned she and her husband were good friends with the Chief and his wife. In fact, they vacationed together every year.

This was valuable information, and I knew that this social networking opportunity could not hurt my job chances after I left town.

My interview with the Chief, the other staff podiatrist and a nurse practitioner went well by all accounts. I left the San Diego VA by 3pm, and flew back to Great Falls that evening. After landing in Great Falls at 11pm, I then had a two-hour drive back to Browning. Needless to say, I was tired.

About a week after my self-funded interview, the official posting appeared on the USAJOBS website. I know from past experience that the government will pay for personal interviews for serious candidates at this level. I was annoyed that I had to pay my own way, even though the secretary told me before my trip that there was no money in the budget for interviews. Apparently, the Chief had plenty of local interest in the job from an ad he placed in the San Diego Podiatric Medical Association Bulletin (where Jeff first learned about the job), but did not have a suitable local candidate.

Weeks went by but the Chief kept stringing me along. During one phone call, he said, "Everyone liked you at the interview, but I need to review the fresh batch of applications I received from the official job posting. My secretary thought you were great."

Meanwhile, Jackson was clearly interested, and I was anxious to rejoin Linda and work again for the VA. In my final conversation with the Chief, he said,

"I have another candidate I like as well as you but I cannot make a decision."

At that point, I was weary of his indecisiveness and had the offer from Jackson. I said, "I'll make it easy for you, I've decided to go to Jackson."

He wished me well, and said; "Now you're one of us."

He never actually offered me the job, and I took the "bird in hand" position in Jackson.

I knew that if the decision were up to the secretary, I would have been offered the position.

Having run my own private practice for nineteen years in Ithaca, whenever I interviewed someone I liked for a job in my office, I acted immediately. Of course, I would always check references first before offering the job. At his request, I faxed the Chief seven recent letters of personal recommendation from my files. I can only speculate at this point why the Chief did not offer me the job in San Diego.

Did he feel threatened by my similar age and experience? During the interview, he kept repeating, "I am the Chief and boss, although I know I need help with various administrative matters."

That job required considerable driving to outlying VA clinics in the San Diego area. I knew from my New Mexico experience that driving, especially though heavy city traffic would quickly wear me out and the cost of living in San Diego was high.

I am convinced now that working for him would have been unpleasant even though the location, climate and proximity to old friends were very seductive.

The one red flag that kept haunting me during this time was that the Chief had some of the same mannerisms as IS.

Is there a personality disorder among VA podiatrists that was indigenous to Southern California?

The process of appointment to Jackson was a harrowing experience. Doctors who work in any accredited hospital in the U.S., VA or otherwise must be properly investigated and credentialed. Prior to Jackson, I had been on staff of thirteen other hospitals, including two Army hospitals and one Indian Health Service hospital. I am squeaky clean professionally, except for the successful conclusion to my malpractice trial. Nevertheless, the process at Jackson was excruciating and unnecessary. The credentialing office in Jackson actually called the Cortland County

(NY) Court to check on my malpractice case, to see if my answer to question #33 on the VA Form 10-2850 was honest.

I had two hurdles to jump before showing up for work there. One was credentialing, where all my education, experience, training, etc. had to be formally verified. The other was the VA Podiatry Board in Cleveland, Ohio that would set my pay level. This Board had previously set my pay at Chief Grade (the highest) prior to my working at the Albuquerque VA, but they had to meet again to determine my pay grade. This is a perfect example of government inefficiency. How could I somehow become less qualified and less experienced while in continuous practice in the government system since 2001? To complicate matters, this Board only met monthly. If all the paperwork from the local VA was not ready, one has to wait until the next month's meeting or until the paperwork was complete.

Of course, you cannot have a formal job offer without a determined salary level. You also cannot apply for a mortgage with a hiring letter that gives a range of salary until the next Board meeting determines your actual pay grade. This greatly complicated our house-hunting task, as we did not really know what our price range would be. We wasted much time looking at less expensive homes due to the salary level uncertainty.

I was originally offered the Jackson position at a much lower salary than I was earning in Browning. I told the Surgical Service Chief I would not consider his offer unless he hired me at Chief Grade. He agreed to my terms, but nothing was finalized on paper. This was equivalent to my previous pay grade at the Albuquerque VA.

For some reason, Jackson was fixated on my starting work on the day after Labor Day. Pay periods in the government are every two weeks, and formally begin on alternate Sundays. If you miss one start day, you have to wait another two weeks to start work. The movers left Montana on August 31st with my household goods and car.

I was homeless and stranded on an Indian reservation without transportation for two weeks.

The government-contracted movers required several weeks' notice to schedule our move from Montana and Texas. The original plan was for me to vacate my government quarters on August 31st, and fly to Texas over that Labor Day weekend. We would drive from our home in Harker Heights, Texas to Jackson, close on our new house on my first day of work the following Tuesday. Our Texas home was to be emptied by that weekend, with our household goods in transit from both locations to our new home in Madison, Mississippi, an upscale suburb of Jackson.

Linda supervised the movers in Texas earlier that week, and I did the same in Browning. The only problem was that I did not officially have a job yet. Most people get a firm job offer and then move. We moved, and then I got the offer.

The Credentials Committee at the Jackson VA was scheduled to review my credentials on Friday morning, August 31st. The Podiatry Board in Cleveland could not rate my pay grade until after the Jackson committee made its decision. At about noon on that Friday, the movers in Montana were about to load my car onto the moving van. I told them,

"Don't load my car onto the van yet."

I certainly did not want my vehicle and half my household goods in Mississippi if I did not have a job there. At 1pm, I finally received a call from credentialing in Jackson that my application had been approved. At that point I said to the movers,

"Ok, load my car onto the van."

They had certainly never heard of such a circumstance before. This left three big problems. I was missing the initial start date, and I did not know how much I was to be paid when I finally did start. I also had to postpone the closing of our new home in Madison originally scheduled for September 4th. My start date was moved up to September 17. Here I was in Browning having moved out of my quarters and with a weekend's worth of belongings in a small suitcase.

I was homeless and car-less on the Blackfeet reservation.

I had to go back to my current employer and extend my job there for two weeks, because a transferring federal employee cannot have a break in service without severe consequences to their future retirement benefits. Meanwhile, Linda and our two dogs had to survive for the two weeks in an empty house with her suitcase, inflatable bed, one pillow (packed several times by the movers after Linda told them not to), one set of dinnerware, and one towel. Fortunately, we kept the major appliances there because we did not know at the time if the Harker Heights house would become rental property.

I moved in with my friend Harold who kept government quarters on the opposite side of the hospital also within walking distance. Neither Linda nor I had TV or a landline telephone, but we had our cell phones. Linda had our Toyota Highlander so she could go grocery shopping.

One of the benefits available to transferring government employees was the home sale program. This allowed the employee a guaranteed home sale to a company designated by the government agency in the event the house does not sell on the open market. This program was established to compete with perks in the private sector. The main caveat was that in order for the employee to enter this program, they are required to live and commute to their last federal job from that home. I was living in government quarters on an Indian reservation, and was obviously not commuting daily from Harker Heights, Texas to Blackfeet Community Hospital in Browning, Montana.

Linda and I spent hours reviewing the GSA regulations regarding this program. Our only recourse was to file an appeal of an initial negative decision to the Civilian Board of Contract Appeals in Washington, D.C. for an exception this rule. We had previously attempted to sell the home and used the two top realtors in the area without success. The real estate market was beginning to fall, as Fort Hood was losing a few Army units to other bases.

A low-level VA employee, citing the rule of needing to live and commute daily from the house to the government job to qualify, denied my initial application to the home sale program. After carefully reviewing all the GSA regulations regarding the government home sale program, I filed my appeal with the Civilian Board of Contract Appeals. The Board was supposed to render a decision within thirty days of filing.

In October, ninety days after moving to Madison and leaving the Harker Heights home empty, we received the judge's decision. She decided not to decide. While the wording of this multi-page decision was favorable, the Board judge ruled that I had a right to have this appeal decided by the proper authority, meaning the Acting Secretary of Veterans Affairs himself. At Linda's insistence, I phoned the office of the Acting VA Secretary Gordon H. Mansfield in Washington, DC.

As Linda suspected, they had not even heard of my case. I immediately faxed all the supporting information, emails, and a copy of the judge's decision to Secretary Mansfield's office. During the first week of December, my contact in his office called me and said that the Secretary himself approved our waiver. Acting Secretary Mansfield was a disabled Vietnam veteran and was impressed with my wife's medical hardships due to the remoteness of the Blackfeet Reservation. I owed him a great debt of gratitude, and we sent him a Christmas card that year.

One of the additional requirements to enter the government home sale program was that the house had to be listed with a Cartus-approved realtor for at least sixty days. Cartus was the company contracted by the government to administer its home sale program. If the house did not sell during that time, Cartus would make a purchase offer as previously described.

Feedback received after one house showing noted that the couple did not like the western exposure of the back patio area. We would have been happy to reorient the house if it was physically possible, but deemed their reason as ridiculous. Other negative comments included a perceived lack of privacy in the back yard. As I mentioned earlier, there was no landscaping in the back yard when we purchased the home three years earlier. The yard sat above the rooftops of the homes on Yak Trail. Without vegetation, we were exposed to the neighbors on Yak.

Linda is an artist, and self-taught landscape architect. She did a masterful job of plantings and has a future vision and imagination lacking in most others. Plants and trees do grow in Texas. We learned from our former neighbors that the house eventually sold, and one of the selling points was the great feeling of privacy in the back yard! Linda's landscape planning and our hard work installing it paid off.

As I mentioned, I had passed the credentials committee in Jackson as I was supervising the loading of my household goods in Montana. We initially arranged for the house closing for September 4th, but without an official letter of hire that included my actual salary, I could not commit to purchasing a home. Through our realtor, I asked our builder to postpone the closing until

September 17th. He agreed, but wanted to charge us and additional sixteen-hundred dollars for his additional "loan costs" due to the two-week delay. Our realtor negotiated this down to one-thousand dollars, as we were financially tapped out from the move.

The builder's father later became my patient at the VA.

We drove from Texas to Jackson and stayed in temporary housing for the few days before the house closing. Monday, September 17 was my first day of work, and also the day of our house closing. The movers were due on the next day.

My new boss, the Chief of Surgical Service at Jackson graciously allowed me the two days off as administrative leave to take care of these important tasks. I just needed to show up for a few hours Monday morning to fill out paperwork to get paid. I could leave after I finished my paperwork.

During that new employee orientation meeting, the Human Resources (HR) official I had been working with the past few months by phone personally sought me out and handed me my official hiring letter that specified my actual salary in writing. It was the first time we met face to face. This was an example of government inefficiency at its worst, and was unnecessarily stressful beyond belief.

My leave status at the Indian Health Service was improperly calculated. I was an hourly employee there, and my timekeeper kept manual records of my hours and leave. I was owed some back leave due to a change in my records from not receiving proper credit for being a former government employee in Albuquerque. Her records were not accurate, and she thought I had more leave owed than the electronic records indicated. The bottom line was that I had to take leave without pay to travel from Browning to Texas and then to Jackson because of the poorly administered IHS record keeping. This was humiliating and expensive.

From July through December, the Texas house stayed empty, and not on the real estate market. Cartus was also the company the government used for its employee relocation services in addition to the home sale program. They had strict guidelines regarding the home sale program, and we did not want to risk violating them. Finally, Cartus purchased our home for the lower of two average appraised values. We lost money on the sale, but were relieved of the headache of long-distance ownership and the financial burdens of owning two homes. We also just made it under the wire before the suspension of this program. Again, we owed a huge debt of gratitude to then-Acting Secretary Mansfield.

Chapter Six

Mississippi, The Magnolia State

aka The Fattest, Poorest, Least, Most...State

2007-2012

Prior to my site visit to the Jackson VA, I had never set foot in Mississippi. I was probably as jaded a northerner as anyone regarding my attitude towards the state. As my plane approached the Jackson area, I could see the Mississippi River as the plane flew over it. The landscape appeared flat, but there were miles of forested land below, speckled with creeks and lakes. I half expected to land in a swamp with snakes and alligators biting at the airplane's wheels.

Upon my arrival at the Jackson-Evers International Airport, there were no reptiles to greet my plane. Instead, I was surprised at the surrounding pine forests and lush vegetation compared to my recent Montana surroundings. I arranged to arrive a full day before my site visit so I could explore the region on my own.

In Browning, I worked with a family doctor named Chad who had moved to the Jackson area about six months before to be near his girlfriend. Aside from working together, we also spent quite a bit of time cross-country and downhill skiing during our off-duty time. Chad was a young member of the "Young and Restless" club. I called Chad and we arranged to meet for dinner just prior to my official site visit. Chad missed the mountain west, and was in limbo with his girlfriend. He was about to give his three-month notice to leave the medical group he was with to return to the Northwest. In Browning, Chad referred me all his patients who required foot surgery and was quite comfortable with that arrangement. At dinner, I asked, "Which podiatrists do you refer to here?"

He replied, "My group refers all foot surgery to orthopedists."

Right then I knew I was in another world years behind the real one.

I spent the Sunday before my Monday interview driving around, primarily Madison County and the Ross Barnett reservoir area. I was quite impressed with the affluence and abundance of nice homes. I even went to several realtor open houses.

My site visit was a carefully scripted event and just happened to coincide with the vacation of the current full-time podiatrist. I reported to the Surgical Service at the VA on a hot June day, dressed in a dark suit. I was under the impression that this visit was still an interview. I was handed an itinerary with appointments to speak with various physician members of the Surgery Department. The Chief of Surgical Service, whom I shall refer to as C-Squared, took me out to lunch. That day, he was uncharacteristically dressed in business casual attire due to the hot weather. After lunch, I met with several more members of the department, including one of the doctors who interviewed me by telephone. All during this time, I kept wondering about the missing podiatrist, and why my visit was scheduled around her leave. It seemed strange to me that my potential future colleague was absent. When I asked about her, I was given vague information. I was told she was very interested in wound care, but that was about all they would say about her. I asked to see the podiatry clinic and was taken to inspect that area.

My final appointment at the end of the day was with C-Squared, where we summarized the day's events. At that point, I was not sure where things stood regarding the job, so I asked, "What happens now?"

He replied, "If you want the job, it's yours."

I said, "Yes, I accept the position."

Apparently, they decided on me immediately after the telephone interview. If I had known that, I would have dressed more comfortably. It was about six pm, and I called Linda as soon as I was outside the front door to deliver the news. She was very happy to hear we would be reunited again after our long separation.

You already know what it took in Chapter Five from the time C-Squared said, "The job is yours if you want it" to actually reporting as a paid employee several months later.

My absent colleague had been working at the Jackson VA for about a year and a half prior to my start.

She was the first full-time podiatrist ever at the hospital and did not have surgical privileges. In fact, I was told up front during my phone interview that surgical privileges were not presently available and might never be. I thought long and hard about that and concluded that I had been performing podiatric surgery for thirty years. If I had to hang up my surgical tools, I could live with it. In reality, I could not. Podiatry is a surgical profession.

I suppose there are many analogies one can use, but imagine a lawyer who regularly tries cases in a courtroom being prevented from doing that. What about a carpenter who has his hammer and saw taken away from him? Ironically, the hospital bylaws were amended to include the requirement that all podiatrists had to have completed at least a two-year surgical residency to be hired. This was an awkward requirement for a podiatrist who would not be granted surgical privileges.

I was educated at a time when two-year podiatric surgical residencies were rare. The American Podiatric Medical Association unofficially recognized the four years I spent in the Army as a podiatrist as the equivalent of this training at the time. I just don't have a piece of paper to show this. The Chief of Staff waved the residency requirement for me in lieu of my Board Certification in foot and ankle surgery, my vast experience, and a telephone call with a former Army podiatrist colleague in Seattle confirming my abilities.

After working for several months, I found myself frustrated at the lack of surgical privileges. We had to refer our podiatric surgical cases to the orthopedists, who were less than thrilled about doing our surgical work. Of course, like many political or administrative decisions in medicine it is ultimately the patient who gets short changed. General orthopedists are competent surgeons, but they just do not perform many of the same specialized procedures we do as podiatric surgeons.

After about a year, the old Director of this VA hospital was replaced. The new Director was a former nurse, and my colleague had worked with her as a podiatry resident at a VA in Alabama. Shortly after the new Director's arrival, we were summoned to the Chief of Staff's office for a meeting with him, C-Squared, the Chief of Staff, and the Assistant Chief of Medicine.

We were told that surgical privileges for podiatrists would be granted immediately. After working out the details of operating room schedules and who would be responsible for the preoperative history and physical exams, with typical government inefficiency I began operating five months after that meeting. I had no doubt that the new Director lit a fire under the behinds of the Chief of Staff and my boss, the Chief of Surgical Service; both of whom I knew had an archaic view of podiatry.

* * *

Living in Mississippi

What was it like for two northerners who love the west to live in Mississippi? As soon as the moving trucks finished unloading our household goods, our new neighbors crossed the street and introduced themselves. Gene asked, "Have Y'all joined a church yet?"

Linda and I were unprepared for that question, so I simply responded, "We really haven't had time to investigate that yet."

Mississippi had been recognized as the most religious state, with over 85% of its polled residents stating that religion was very important in their lives. We thought Texas was religious, but here religion was flagrantly displayed. We had never before encountered more Christian bumper stickers or front license plate signs. The neighbors across the street had a wrought iron cross attached to the brick front of their house. Southern Baptist Sunday services last the better part of the day and many also attend services on Wednesday evenings. (We enjoyed having the development's outdoor pool to ourselves on summer Sunday mornings – except when the water moccasins were swimming there!)

The state was also the fattest (greatest number of obese residents), the poorest, and the state with the least number of adults with bachelor's degrees. It was tempting to call Mississippians fat, dumb, and happy. That characterization would really not be fair. (Unfortunately, as of this recent editing, New Mexico has replaced Mississippi as having the worst public education system in the country). Mississippi is home to the University Medical Center and medical school where the world's first heart transplant was performed. Mississippi State University has a veterinary college that provided exceptional care to our late beloved female Shih Tzu, Gisele. She would have died there if not for the care she received at the school. Montana has neither a medical nor a veterinary school.

Mississippi is the home of Blues music, Elvis Presley, and is the home state of famous authors William Faulkner, Eudora Welty, John Grisham, Greg Iles, and James Dickerson. This is also the home state of Morgan Freeman and Oprah Winfrey. Brett Favre, Archie Manning, and his sons Peyton and Eli, Jerry Rice and the late Steve McNair played college football here. All this being said, when the weekend arrived, Linda and I were hard pressed to find things to do. We were accustomed to outdoor activity such as hiking, sightseeing and water sports. The Ross Barnett reservoir was a local resource, but I did not relish kayaking in alligator and snake infested waters. I needed both hands for my work.

Hunting and fishing in Mississippi ranked close to religion. Montana is known for world class hunting and fishing, but here it was fully integrated into the fabric of the local culture. Exclusive deer camps, hunting and fishing lodges abounded, and some people paid small fortunes to belong to duck hunting clubs. Four-wheeled ATVs were more common than bicycles in our housing development. My patients often asked me, "Doc, do you hunt or fish?"

"I used to, but now I can afford to buy my meat and fish at the grocery store."

This smart-ass remark covered up the real reason I gave up those sports. I have become soft in my old age. Owning dogs has made me compassionate in regards to the suffering and pain of animals. I would hunt and fish for survival, but no longer for sport.

Jackson is the capital city of the state and its largest city. After consulting with others, we purchased a home in Madison. This was an upscale suburb with the best schools in the state and an easy commute to the VA.

One of the many reasons we left Montana was due to the severity of the winters for Linda. The summers in Mississippi were hot and humid, and sapped the energy from our bodies. The winters can be cold, with nighttime temperatures below freezing on some nights. We've had a dusting of snow for one day during each winter. One February day, however, we had 5 inches of snow. Linda said, "Let's get out our cross-country skis."

My good friend Harold made me a ski rack from old barn wood from his ranch. Of course, that moved with the rest of our household items including pairs of cross country and downhill skis. The ski rack loaded with skis was out of place in a Mississippi garage, but that day we put our equipment to good use. We drove to a nearby golf course, which are popular places to cross country ski in snow country and donned our skis. People stopped their cars to watch us. I thought about contacting the Jackson newspaper, but decided I really did not want the notoriety. I have no doubt we were the only ones in Mississippi to ski on that day. We took photos.

We had great fun.

In spite of our few moments of fun in the snow, we were both happy to be out of the northeast's unforgiving winter weather.

Unlike private practice or other VAs, I had no choice in the selection of my colleague. Nor did she with me. My memory is not clear about when I first met her, but I recall a conversation with the podiatry nurse, Charlene, regarding her prior to our initial meeting. I'll refer to my colleague as DQ for this chapter. The "D" does not stand for "Dairy."

My "D" stands for "Drama." It was either that title or CL for "Chicken Little," as nearly every activity in her life was either some monumental event was about to take place in her life or the sky was falling.

Charlene told me that DQ was going through a divorce and that her husband, Bill, was also a podiatrist practicing in Alabama. It seems that DQ got involved in an affair with her VA Director in Alabama. Robert was originally from Mississippi, and I suspect was somehow instrumental in getting DQ the position in Jackson. The plan was they would see each other at his Mississippi farm on weekends and go to their respective work places during the week. Bill and DQ had an eight-year-old daughter.

DQ was an attractive blond who was passionate about treating wounds. This was good for me professionally because I was not really up to speed with that rapidly advancing subspecialty of podiatry. We complemented each other with our different skill sets and strengths; mine in elective podiatric surgery and nerve conditions of the foot and hers in wound care. We worked together for three years until she left for another VA position in Central Florida to be near her family. I spent a year-and-a-half as the only podiatrist at the Jackson VA after she left. I took wound care to new heights, employing new modalities that surpassed her treatments. She was never one to give direct compliments, but I heard from one of our wound care product company reps that she learned from me also.

She was difficult to work with.

Every day there was either some new conspiracy or legal proceeding she was involved with. I tried to listen politely without being drawn into the fray. Linda eventually forbid me from telling her about the daily drama when I came home from work. DQ often spoke in conspirational whispers that I had a difficult time hearing.

It reminded me of being back in public school and I felt that her actions were very immature.

At first, I believed her that she and Bill were splitting, and that she and Robert had a future.

It turned out that Bill was just closing up his practice in Alabama so he could move back to Madison, MS to be with DQ and their daughter. It seemed to me that she wanted it both ways; a husband and family and a boyfriend. When I finally met Bill, I wondered what he thought about their situation and how he permitted the situation to continue. As I got to know him better, I found him to be equally disingenuous.

Robert got into administrative trouble and was forced into retirement. That coincided with the end of their affair. I never met him. DQ was both an Army veteran like me and then joined the Navy before going to podiatry school. She was beginning the process of joining the Naval Reserves, and I had to fill out some paperwork for that on her behalf. As far as I know, she never followed through with it.

Both of us were professionally unhappy at Jackson, and we were both looking to leave there.

Our boss, C-Squared, was trained as a general surgeon who had not operated for at least ten years. He came to work every day (except for the day of my site visit) in a starched shirt and bow tie. He surrounded himself with five secretaries and stayed either in his office or in meetings. He never once, in the four-and-a-half years I worked there, visited the podiatry clinic. His superiors forced podiatry upon him, but he maintained his dinosaur opinion of the profession.

When an experienced surgeon arrives at a new duty station, it is not unusual for him/her to introduce at least one new procedure to the existing staff. As I previously wrote, I introduced the Fort Hood podiatrists to the EPF procedure.

I became friendly with Lloyd Martin, MD. Lloyd was an orthopedic surgeon. Aside from our similar professional interests, Lloyd and I shared some common experiences. He grew up in Albuquerque and was also an Army veteran. As a young Army orthopedist, he was stationed at Fort Benning, Georgia. Fort Benning is home to the Army's airborne training center and fractured ankles are common from bad parachute landings. Soon after his arrival, Lloyd announced to the Chief of Podiatry there that he would fix all the broken ankles. George Gilman, DPM, was Chief of the Podiatry Section. George was also my podiatry school classmate. He told Lloyd, "I fix all the broken ankles around here."

Few surgeons in the world had surgically repaired more broken ankles than George. He had authored a textbook on that subject and lectured extensively at professional meetings. Lloyd did a lot of assisting for George.

There is some overlap with orthopedics and podiatry. After completing a four-year orthopedic residency, a graduating resident can elect to go on to a one-year fellowship in one of the various orthopedic subspecialties or go into practice as a general orthopedist. One of the fellowship programs is in foot and ankle surgery. The main difference in orthopedic fellowship training in foot and ankle surgery and podiatry training is that podiatric residencies in foot and ankle surgery are for three years beyond podiatry school.

One of the promises I was made by C-Squared when he interviewed me, was that there would be an academic affiliation for me with the University of Mississippi (UMC) medical school, across the street from the VA. That never happened in spite of the fact that the incidence of lower limb amputations in Mississippi from diabetes was one of the highest in the US. UMC desperately needed podiatrists on their staff to complete a limb salvage team, as exist at places like Georgetown University, the University of Arizona, and the University of Southern California.

I wrote a letter to the Chief of Staff of UMC, along with an evidenced based article demonstrating the positive effect podiatrists have as part of a team to save limbs (and therefore save lives).

I never received a response.

Lloyd watched me perform an EPF procedure, and he liked it. He said to me,

"Evan, I have a senior resident who is going to a foot and ankle fellowship in a few months. Would you mind if he scrubbed in on your next case?"

Having trained podiatric residents before at the Albuquerque VA, I was pleased to do so.

The following Friday, the resident assisted me in my EPF case. On the following Monday, I received a nasty email from my boss, C-Squared, telling me I could not be involved in training residents as I had no affiliation with UMC. Furthermore, he went on to say that podiatrists were not permitted to train orthopedic surgeons. You do remember what the Chief of Orthopedics at the Albuquerque VA told me. Years before when I was in the Army at Fort Meade, Maryland, I showed two Navy orthopedists from the US Naval Academy in nearby Annapolis how to perform a particular bunion surgery.

I was furious and highly insulted. I said to Lloyd, "You asked me to do this. Would you please speak to our boss about this?" During the meeting, Lloyd told me that C-Squared was unwavering in his position, even if Lloyd himself were in the operating room with a resident and me.

The overall Chief of Podiatry in the VA system who worked in Cleveland, Ohio told me something which did help mollify my feelings, he said, "Evan, people who are insecure themselves often feel threatened by situations such as this. You should really feel sorry for them."

If I had artistic ability, I would draw a caricature of C-Squared sitting as a skeleton at his computer with his bow tie hanging from his cervical spine and cobwebs hanging from his humeral bones.

Hopefully you can picture this without the benefit of my crude drawing.

He should have retired years ago.

I was always cordial and respectful to C-Squared, and he mostly treated me in kind. In spite of this incident, I always received outstanding evaluations from him across the board for my four annual performance appraisals. (Remember the evaluation from the Albuquerque VA). I appreciated him for that.

DQ and C-Squared did not get along. She was well versed in VA rules and regulations, as her residency director in Alabama taught her the ropes in that regard. She was always filing official complaints against C-Squared, the Chief of Staff, and others. I refused to be drawn into those disputes.

On a Monday before Christmas week, DQ came to work like any other Monday. On Tuesday, she announced she was leaving on Thursday. I was not surprised she was leaving, but was angry at the way she did it. Without any consideration for her colleague (me), I now had to see all the patients by myself. By doing it her way, she selfishly avoided any personal discomfort often experienced by departing employees during the typical "two-week notice period". She instituted what she called the "KMA" procedure, aka "Kiss My Ass" as she walked out the door for the last time.

I would never pull a stunt like that on another colleague.

I am certainly not a psychiatrist, but I believe DQ suffered from a potentially treatable mental disorder. She was otherwise bright and capable and with proper treatment I believed she could have been a much better person. She also displayed a stunning lack of personal commitment to just about everything; her marriage, future Navy career, her colleague, and even to her own profession.

There was another clinic adjacent to the Podiatry Clinic. It was called the Lower Extremity Clinic, and run by a nurse practitioner I'll call EB, short for "Evil Bitch." She was a wannabe podiatrist without a fraction of the training, knowledge or skills.

When I first arrived at the Jackson VA, we were friendly to each other. She wanted me to teach her some of my skills. DQ warned me that that could be dangerous to patients, since EB did not have the medical knowledge to safely administer some of those treatments. EB also treated lower extremity wounds, and performed what podiatrists refer to as "C and C." This refers to the routine trimming of toenails, corns and calluses.

As I have mentioned, we were without surgical privileges for the first year I was there. There were two part-time contract podiatrists who only worked Wednesday mornings, doing mostly C and C work. They made a fortune at this as contractors, ripping off the government in my opinion, and were poor examples of what podiatrists are capable of. The new director correctly terminated their contract.

After about six months into my new job, EB realized I was not going to show her anything.

One day, she made a very insulting and totally inaccurate remark regarding my professional skills, and I immediately went to her boss to file a complaint.

For the remaining four years of my time there, we never spoke to each other after that incident.

It was not for these reasons I call her EB. I hope I rose above her level.

For some reason unknown to me, she disliked one of our company reps, John. He was an outgoing and good-looking family man with two young boys who was about the same age as DQ. EB started a false rumor that John and DQ were having an affair. That vicious rumor began the unraveling of John's marriage. Since EB also disliked DQ (maybe jealousy), she created another nasty rumor about an alleged affair between DQ and another surgeon. Fortunately, that went nowhere and to my knowledge harmed no one. EB enjoyed starting these rumors and always looked for ways to mind other people's business. She was understandably considered a toxic person and shunned by most of the other professional staff. Unfortunately, the Government protected her and many others like her with layers of rules and regulations preventing them from being fired.

Mississippi was the most obese state, with West Virginia a close second. It was not uncommon to walk the halls of the Jackson VA and pass by people who exceeded 400 pounds. They would lumber along, completely oblivious to their surroundings. They lacked what I call, "kinesthetic awareness," or the sense of their body movements in space and time. This is something I've developed from my many years of skiing and my brief exposure to the martial arts. As I passed by these huge people, men and women alike, it was almost as if I could feel a gravitational pull from their massive bodies.

Holmes County, just north of Madison County, boasted the nation's shortest lifespan for men, at 66 years (NPR, June 17, 2011). I do not know the location of the US County with the greatest longevity, but the life span for men there was fifteen years longer (NPR, June 17, 2011).

Aside from my "Arthur" patient whom you met in the Introduction, I had other memorable patient interactions at the Jackson VA. Dr. Comfort is a company that makes diabetic footwear. The company promoted its products at professional podiatry conferences by having a display booth in the vendor area. The sales representatives who were staffing the booth at one meeting I attended were giving away plastic shoe horns with their name, "Dr. Comfort" prominently displayed in gold paint on the handle of the item.

As a courtesy to my patients, I always had a shoe horn available to make it easier for them to don their shoes after their treatment was completed. One day, as a patient was putting on his shoes using my Dr. Comfort shoe horn, he asked me, "Are you Dr. Comfort?" Apparently, I hadn't properly introduced myself, so I replied, "Why don't you tell me after you stand up and walk around."

Another memorable encounter occurred when I asked a new patient, "What brings you to the clinic today?" He replied, "I have a farmer's wart." I said, "I'm not familiar with that." He said, "You know doc, a planter's wart." I said, "You mean a plantar's wart." A wart on the bottom, or plantar aspect of the foot is what he meant.

As a sad testament to the often poorly educated veterans in Mississippi, a patient asked me what I knew to be a serious question from him: "Doc, what's a calorie?"

With my physical science and teaching background, I proceeded to explain to him the physics and chemistry definition of that term and related it to food and nutrition. He seemed to understand my descriptions and was very grateful for my explanation.

I also had the honor and privilege to treat Easy Thigpen (real name!) a 90+ year-old who was one of the last surviving members of the Tuskegee Airmen of World War Two fame. That year, the remaining survivors were being honored in Washington with a fully paid for trip to D.C. Unfortunately, Mr. Thigpen was not able to attend due his poor health.

One other final fact about the Jackson VA was that it was named after G.V. (Sonny) Montgomery. He was a long-serving congressman from the state who was a Major General in the Mississippi National Guard and the author of the first G.I. Bill of Rights.

My exit strategy for leaving the Jackson VA was similar to Montana. Fortunately, I had a nice large, private office with a window.

Having committed to retiring from a government career, I checked the USAJOBS website on a daily basis. I really wanted to get back into teaching residents like I did in Albuquerque, but I would have willingly taken another podiatrist job in a better location than Jackson. I applied to several jobs, one for the Chief of Podiatry position at the brand-new VA hospital in Las Vegas. Linda had cousins who live there and we went to visit them. Linda had not seen them since childhood and they were very nice people.

Chapter Seven

Return to Texas, The Alamo City

2012-2018

There was a non-government job posting for an academic position in San Antonio, Texas. This was with the University of Texas Health Science Center, Division of Podiatric Medicine and Surgery, Department of Orthopedics. In doing my research, I learned that this was a job paid by the State of Texas. If I worked for the state for at least five years, I could retire with a pension. Since I was eligible to retire from the VA at any time, this was an appealing opportunity to have two pensions.

I've always liked San Antonio, having spent some time there while in the Army and during visits. Texas was a good state for retirees, and San Antonio has a better winter climate than Jackson. I also researched salaries for assistant professorships at medical schools. The median income was higher than my VA salary.

I went to San Antonio on a self-paid interview trip. The afternoon interview went well. I got along with everyone whom I would be working with. I stayed until the next morning, which was the start of a professional conference. I was able to socialize with my potential future colleagues before the meeting, and one let it slip, saying, "I'll see you in a few months."

I did not sign up or pay to attend the meeting, so I left to catch my plane. A week later the head of the department called and offered me the job. This would have been my dream job; an academic position at a prestigious medical school. The only problem was that Texas, like many other states, was having financial difficulties. The salary was actually considerably lower than my current VA salary. I could not responsibly accept that position for lower pay at this stage in my life. I was disappointed.

About nine months later, a VA job was posted in, you guessed it; San Antonio. Podiatry residents from the program I declined also rotated through the VA. I realized that if I applied and were chosen for this position, I would be training the same residents but at my current salary. There was also promise of an academic affiliation with the University.

I filed my formal application in October. There was an upcoming VA-wide podiatry conference in Phoenix I was planning to attend, and I was fairly certain the Chief of Podiatry at the San Antonio VA would be there. I wrote him a letter expressing my interest in the position and hoped I could meet him personally.

I met him there and introduced myself. I knew he was a wound care expert, and I presented a challenging case of a patient I had in Jackson. I asked his advice regarding treatment, which he freely gave. He also said, "I received your application and you will be getting a phone call to set up a phone interview."

That was the extent of our personal interaction at the conference. A week after I returned to Jackson, I participated in the phone interview with two other members of the surgical staff. One was Brad Hardy, MD, who was the Chief of Surgical Service.

I did well on the interview, and a week after that, Brad called and offered me the job. This was in mid-December. You already know the steps it takes to bring on a new doctor, even one who transfers from one VA to another. Our government must again reinvent the proverbial wheel.

When Human Resources formally offered me the job, I accepted. The salary was the same as I was already earning in Jackson, but this job posted an incentive and relocation bonus. This time, the government would not pay for their low budget movers, nor was the guaranteed home buyout program available. I would just receive a cash bonus from which I would pay for my own moving expenses. We were on our own in selling our house.

Dr. Hardy told me in a later phone call what he felt the VA would pay as a bonus. I asked him to ask the director for more, since I knew it could be as much as twenty five percent of my salary. He was concerned that if I did not get what I asked for, I would decline the offer. I simply said, "It doesn't hurt to ask. All she can say is no."

Before the Director made her decision on my bonus, HR asked me to fax a copy of my latest performance appraisal to them. C-Squared gave me "outstandings" in all categories.

The Director met my request.

I began the process of credentialing among other tasks.

A few weeks later, as I was well on my administrative way to San Antonio, I received a surprise call from the Chief of Staff at the Las Vegas VA. This caught me completely unprepared, since I had absolutely no contact with them since I had applied nine months ago. He asked, "Dr. Meltzer, are you still interested in the Chief of Podiatry position at our hospital?"

I replied, "I would have been, but I have committed to another VA. What took so long for you to respond to my application?"

I was fed typical government-speak as reasons for their delay. The pay would have been the same, and there was no teaching, but I would have been the boss. It was appealing to work at a new facility and with Linda's family in the area, but I was already committed.

Before leaving Jackson, I had access to all of my VA evaluations. My reaction to seeing my "official" evaluation from Albuquerque was a combination of anger, resentment and irony that JD from Albuquerque had changed his final evaluation of me to all "Satisfactory". In so doing, he saved his government career and created an interesting detour to mine.

In retrospect, however, I'm thankful for his actions that allowed me to serve at Ft. Hood and Browning. This action on JD's part was a good example of how the government corruption can exist at any position level. And besides, this memoir wouldn't even exist, but since it does, please continue reading.

* * *

In January of 2012, I received the following email. It was one of the nicest professional correspondences I had ever received:

Subject: I Hear a Welcome to San Antonio is in Order!

Hello Dr. Meltzer,
"I cannot believe the irony that I was talking about you with our department administrator today and discussing our disappointment on not being able to offer you enough to have you come on board with

us here at the University. And just now, this afternoon, our residency director, Michael Park, DPM, tells me he talked with the VA Chief of Podiatry and informed him you are coming to the VA in San Antonio.

We are thrilled to hear that! We know you have a lot to offer and if we could not get you to join us at the University this is the next best thing. We look forward to your arrival and seeing you once again. Please stop by to see us once you are in town."

Sincerely, Business Administrator
Division of Podiatric Medicine & Surgery
Department of Orthopaedics
University of Texas Health Science Center at San Antonio.

In summary, I did receive an appointment as an Adjunct Assistant Professor at the UT Health Sciences Center at San Antonio, fulfilling a life-long professional dream of being a professor at a prestigious institution such as the University of Texas. There was no additional pay with the title "Adjunct", but all other privileges of the regular faculty are accorded such as University library access, etc. I enjoyed working with the young residents.

The patients at the Audie L. Murphy VA Hospital in San Antonio were the sickest patients I had ever treated, including the patients I saw on the Indian reservations previously discussed. Whether it was the Hispanic culture and associated diet or some other influence on their attitude, many of the diabetic patients didn't seem to care about their health. They wanted to live their lives as they wished and expected us to fix their problems. You must know that we are not miracle workers!

I also worked closely with an Infectious Disease physician. We shared many of the same patients, where he treated their infections with the appropriate antibiotics and I would do the surgical care such as weekly debridement of their wounds. He would often ask us to call him when a particularly at-risk patient was in our clinic, and he would come over from his clinic to check on the patient's progress or regress. We learned from each other.

The podiatry residents took turns being on-call 24/7, rotating between the VA and the University, as residents cannot operate unsupervised. With three other attending podiatrists at the VA to share the load, we would each spend one week per month on-call. During our week on-call, we would frequently be called by the resident-on-call at all hours of the night to discuss emergent and non-emergent cases. In several instances, we would have to go to the Hospital in the middle of the night to perform an emergency surgery. What constitutes an emergency surgery in podiatric medicine you may ask? Gas gangrene or a severe abscess that requires an emergent incision and drainage to prevent sepsis and death in that particular patient represents a surgical emergency. Many of these patients progressed to partial foot amputations, which we did, or to a higher level of amputation below or above the knee performed by our orthopedic or general surgical colleagues. I had never before done more partial foot amputations in my other previous positions as I had done at this VA.

Podiatry also worked in close association with the vascular surgery department. No wound can heal without adequate blood flow. There is a particular test called the non-invasive vascular study. This test provides results that doctors can use to predict whether or not a diabetic foot wound has a good chance of healing or not. In some cases, the vascular surgeons would need to operate first to restore proper circulation to the affected lower extremity before we would get involved in their wound care.

I was fortunate to share an office for five years with Dr. Marvin Martinez, a San Antonio native. He was very smart and we would often discuss our cases with each other. Sometimes he had to remind me that I forgot to order the vascular study described above on a particular patient. We learned from each other. I was also fortunate to have two other bright colleagues, Sean and Frank, who was the Chief of the department I had originally met in Phoenix. Their combined collegiality was a vast improvement over DQ and EB at the Jackson VA.

Not to be left out of the team who treats diabetics is the patient's primary care doctor. That professional is supposed to be the "Captain of the Ship", who ideally knows and coordinates all his/her patient's appointments with these specialists. I must also mention the specialty of endocrinology or diabetology for certain patients whose underlying disease process is difficult to control. Nutritional, life-style education and exercise options are also available in the VA system.

The beauty and patient safety aspect of the VA medical system is that every treating provider has access to the patient's complete medical records including all medications and all notes from all of his providers. I say "his" because of all the veterans I treated with diabetic foot wounds, only two were female! As you can see, the treatment of the diabetic foot is a multi-disciplinary task, and in 2012, when I left Jackson, the University of Mississippi Medical School really did their diabetic foot patients a disservice by not including podiatry (America's true foot and ankle specialists) in the treatment of that subset of patients. I finally decided that at age seventy-two, being on-call became too much, and I retired in 2018 and Linda and I returned to New Mexico.

Returning to The Land of Enchantment continues to bring us pleasure, and Linda again has the opportunity to design a new landscape and vegetable garden in this high desert region. I've rejoined her effective and exclusive "Work-Hardening Program" but am able to bike in the warm months when I am not digging holes for planting and downhill skiing not far from home in the winter.

I hope you have enjoyed sharing this adventure with me and learned a few things about my profession and the trials and tribulations experienced by some "rich doctors".

* * *

Chapter Eight

Final Thoughts

As you now know from reading my memoir, I spent half of my professional career in private practice and the other half in what I call "public practice." I believe I am uniquely qualified to comment on both models of medical practice.

To succeed in private practice, one must have at least these three attributes: The first is knowledge and skill in one's chosen medical field. The second is business savvy, and the third is having a good bedside manner or otherwise known as a pleasant personality. Another very helpful trait to have is the intuitive skill to decide exactly what the patient is expecting during their encounter. Are they seeking your empathy and just treatment of their problem or are they someone who can enjoy a bit of humor?

I had a patient at the Audie Murphy VA Medical Center in San Antonio who I treated conservatively for a diabetic wound on his right second toe (the toe next to the big toe). After some weeks of treatment it became clear to both of us that conservative care would not heal this chronic wound. After discussing with him his options, he agreed to have me amputate the toe. The resulting surgical wound healed uneventfully and when he came to see me for his final post operative visit, there was a tattoo facing me just proximal to the empty space where his toe was that said, "Stayed Home." Those of you who remember the children's nursery rhyme, "This Little Piggy…" will understand!

I believe that any practitioner in private practice will not succeed if they are missing one or more of these traits.

I was in private solo practice for the nineteen years of my various practice experiences. The solo practice model is becoming more uncommon in today's American medical world. Although you may be the boss and take vacation whenever you want, you are responsible for one-hundred percent of office overhead and salary for your employees and you're also the personnel manager. You must also make arrangements for your patients in case of emergency while you are away. Most podiatrists finishing their residencies today opt for joining an existing group practice or become employees of hospitals, or work where I worked. Solo private podiatry practices can still be found.

I became Board Certified in Foot and Ankle Surgery and thus met my first requirement. My late father was self-employed his entire working life. He was my first business consultant. There are also professional business consultants that can be hired. When Linda was the office manager our income was the highest with her in charge of the front desk. I took continuing education courses in marketing, and seriously considered studying for a Masters in Business Administration (MBA) after hours. I had met my second requirement. I maintained a healthy practice in Ithaca that well-supported Linda and me, so I met my third requirement. We were able to take nice vacations to wonderful places and lived in a beautiful house overlooking Cayuga Lake as described in the New York chapter.

In "public practice" one only needs to meet the first requirement of professional competence. As a government-employed provider, business sense and personality usually will not affect one's salary (a charming and obsequious personality towards one's superiors could affect salary and promotion, otherwise known as "kissing ass"). I pointed this out with examples of EB and DQ in Jackson and IS in Albuquerque. There were also similar personalities at the San Antonio VA, who would in my opinion not succeed in private practice. (I am not referring to my former collegues.)

My experience with the VA has shown me that this system attracts both the best and worst providers. The best are those who totally focus on the veteran patient in front of them with the goal of providing the best care possible without having the headaches of managing a private practice. My San Antonio VA colleagues were an excellent example of that model.

The worst are those who focus mainly on their government careers and often place patient care and the welfare of their subordinate employees a distant second to their own goals and egos. It is also my belief that the current VA health care system has far more of the best providers than the worst. It has been my personal experience that I've enjoyed excellent healthcare as a veteran patient at the several VAMC hospitals where I've received my healthcare. Unfortunately, some veteran patients have had poor experiences and have complained about their lack of quality healthcare. I believe that this group may have had exposure to one or more providers of the second kind that I've outlined above and are in the small minority of veteran patients. Every level one VA hospital has a patient advocate office where an unhappy patient may take their complaints to and have their issues resolved.

The VA system may become a future model for universal health care if the powerful health insurance industry can ever be pushed aside for the greater good of all Americans.

* * *

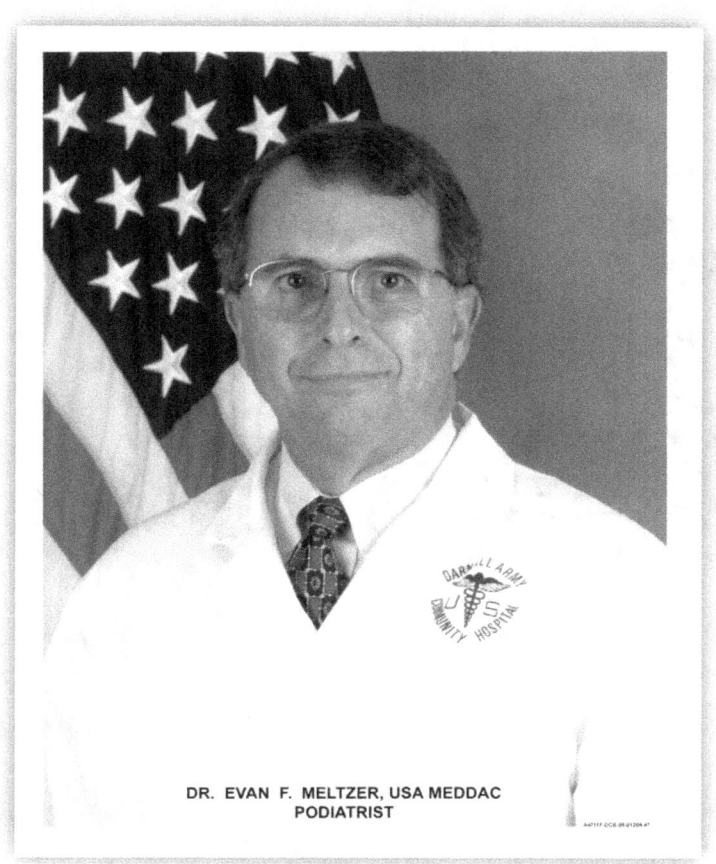

DR. EVAN F. MELTZER, USA MEDDAC
PODIATRIST

ABOUT THE AUTHOR

Dr. Evan Meltzer retired after practicing podiatric medicine and surgery for forty-one years. For half of his professional career, he was in private practice. For the last half of his career, he was an employed podiatrist with the Department of the Army, the Indian Health Service and the Department of Veterans Affairs.

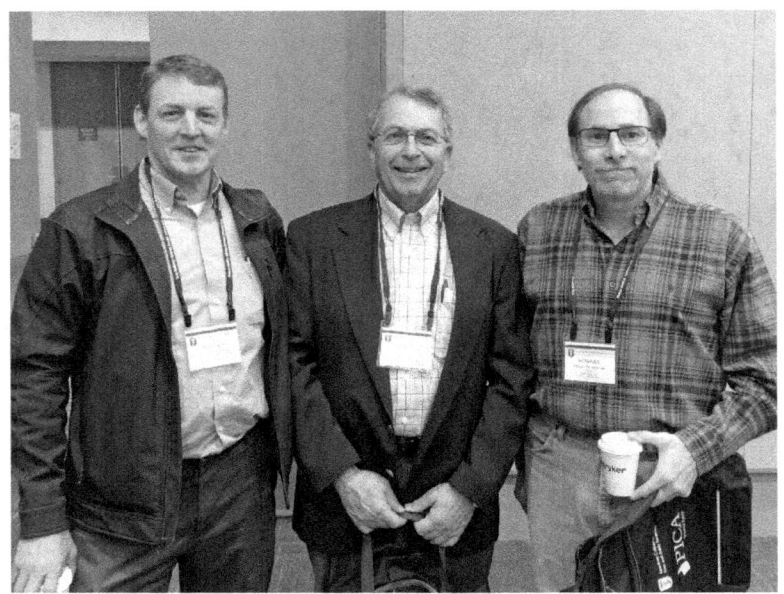

Fort Hood Colleagues

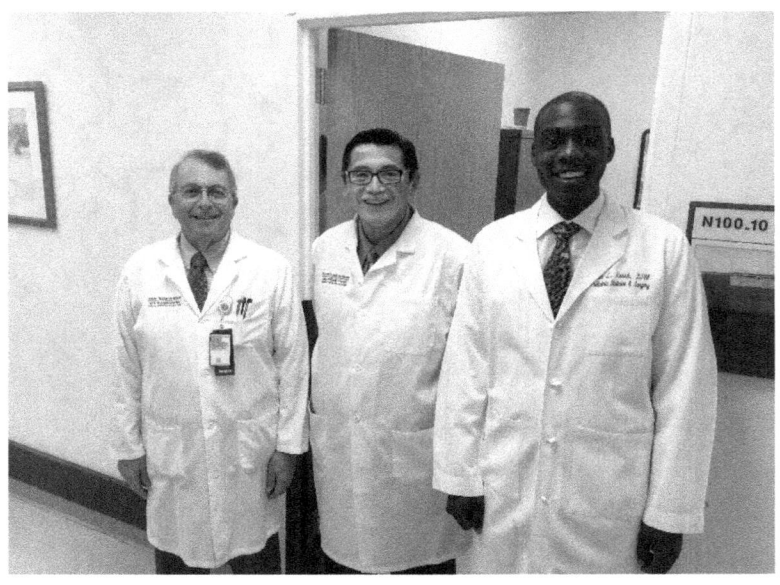

San Antonio VA Colleagues

Acknowledgments

I would like to thank the following individuals who have helped me in many ways by editing my work and providing much appreciated support during this process:

Michael Numan, Ph.D. is a retired professor of neuroscience from Boston College and was my neighbor. Michael read and edited the manuscript. He also suggested that I include the dates of my time spent at each location so the reader can follow with the dates that each chapter covers. He and I have much in common. We both grew up in New York State and are only two months apart in age. We enjoyed taking walks together in our neighborhood.

He and his wife recently moved to California to be near their anesthesiologist daughter. I miss our walks, his intelligence and the similar views of life in general that we shared.

Robert Simmons, Ph.D. and I had initially met in Ithaca when Bob was hosting a men's support group at his apartment for separated and divorced men. Bob is a clinical psychologist who had also been a college professor at Cortland State and commuted there from his home in Ithaca. Bob moved back to his hometown of San Diego after retiring from a government psychology job treating soldiers at Fort Drum near Watertown, NY after leaving Cortland State for that position. He edited my manuscript and was quite helpful with his recommendations. He tells me that he doesn't miss the winters in upstate New York.

Neil Hodges is a college friend and a retired social worker for the State of Michigan and worked in the nearby capital city of Lansing. He lives in Okemos, so close to the Michigan State University campus that he can sometimes hear cheering from Spartan Stadium during football season (although there hasn't been much to cheer about lately). Neil and his wife Mary traveled to Guatemala two decades before me and read my chapter about my experiences there. He asked me to be a bit less critical of that third world country, and I took his advice.

Mark Lanier, DVM was my last roommate in college before my first marriage. He owned successful veterinary practices in the greater Detroit area before retiring to northern Michigan. He has been my "Jimminy Cricket" for years and has gently persuaded me to examine and accept my true religious beliefs.

Robert Valins, DPM was a podiatry school classmate and still a close friend. He reminded me of the advice I gave him some fifty years ago when we were students. I had forgotten what I told him at that time but he reminded me of what I said to him. Bob told me that what I said was to "apply for everything you want and let someone else make the decision." He was so impressed with my advice to him then that he recently applied to me when I was seriously thinking about un-retiring and applying for podiatry jobs.

Although he received a copy of the manuscript, he hasn't had the time to read it. As of this editing he is still working part-time and is trying to conclude a buyout agreement with his partners and retire from the very successful six-doctor podiatry practice that he founded in Tampa, FL in 1978.

I also wish to acknowledge and thank James L. Dickerson of Brandon, Mississippi. He got me started on this path in 2009. Jim is an accomplished and prolific author and literary agent who taught a class I attended at night at Millsaps College in Jackson on "How to Sell What You Write." I had never really thought about publishing a memoir but after he read a sample of my writing, Jim was very encouraging and made many helpful suggestions.

My cousin, Ellen Glicken Brazer, first introduced me to the concept of self-publishing. She has successfully written and self-published five books through KDP-Amazon.

Vicki Fowler, DVM, my longest living lifetime friend. Vicki, a retired veterinarian, has been my friend and classmate from kindergarten through college. From #1 school and East High School in Rochester, NY to Michigan State University, Vicki has always been there for me for moral support and friendly advice.

And finally, Rose Marie Kern. Rose was the instructor of a virtual publishing class I attended offered by the SouthWest Writers of Albuquerque. Rose did the formatting and artistic design along with general editing and moral support for this book.

www.ingramcontent.com/pod-product-compliance
Lightning Source LLC
Chambersburg PA
CBHW052346220526
45465CB00003BA/980